How to Lose Weight with

INTERMITTENT FASTING

The Complete Guide to Safe Fasting, Lose Weight and Rejuvenate with Metabolism Reset.

Bonus:

1) *50 + delicious recipes & meal plan for 4 weeks*
2) *5/2 method and how to combine keto*

| June 2021 Edition |

TABLE OF CONTENT

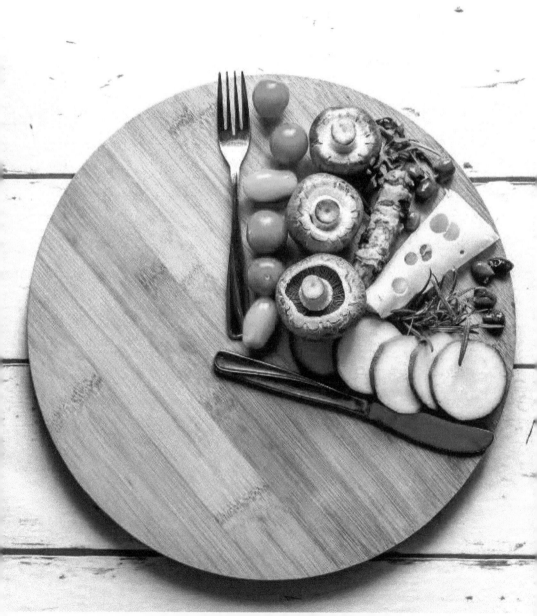

Legal & Disclaimer

The information contained in this book and its contents is not designed to replace or take the place of any form of medical or professional advice; and is not meant to replace the need for independent medical, financial, legal or other professional advice or services, as may be required. The content and information in this book have been provided for educational and entertainment purposes only.

The content and information contained in this book has been compiled from sources deemed reliable, and it is accurate to the best of the Author's knowledge, information and belief. However, the Author cannot guarantee its accuracy and validity and cannot be held liable for any errors and/or omissions. Further, changes are periodically made to this book as and when needed. Where appropriate and/or necessary, you must consult a professional (including but not limited to your doctor, attorney, financial advisor or such other professional advisor) before using any of the suggested remedies, techniques, or information in this book.

Upon using the contents and information contained in this book, you agree to hold harmless the Author from and against any damages, costs, and expenses, including any legal fees potentially resulting from the application of any of the information provided by this book. This disclaimer applies to any loss, damages or injury caused by the use and application, whether directly or indirectly, of any advice or information presented, whether for breach of contract, tort, negligence, personal injury, criminal intent, or under any other cause of action.

You agree to accept all risks of using the information presented inside this book.

You agree that by continuing to read this book, where appropriate and/or necessary, you shall consult a professional (including but not limited to your doctor, attorney, or financial advisor or such other advisor as needed) before using any of the suggested remedies, techniques, or information in this book.

INTRODUCTION

The subject matter "INTERMITTENT FASTING" is a dietary approach and obviously not a new thing to most people but information makes the world go round that is why this book is written for use of every individual across the globe. Most especially, people who are not well informed about the topic of discuss. The primary objective of this book is to make anyone who is interested in engaging in "IF" have self sufficient before embarking on the amazing journey of Intermittent fasting.

This book is written in a friendly manner and by the end of the day when each reader must have feasted on the contents, very reader must have had adequate and self sufficient knowledge about;

- ❖ *What is Intermittent Fasting*
- ❖ *Techniques of intermittent fasting*
- ❖ *The 16/8 method4 step by step*
- ❖ *Potentials Of "IF"*
- ❖ *Intermittent Fasting Hacks*
- ❖ *Intermittent Fasting And The Ketogenic diet*
- ❖ *30 days Intermittent Fasting Meal Plan.*

This book is the door and an ultimate guide to executing an effective 16/8 intermittent fasting which is why it is written in a friendly and comprehensible manner. All you need to know about the 16/8 plan has been documented in this book for your use. Enjoy!

CHAPTER ONE

What is Intermittent Fasting

Intermittent fasting is not a diet, it's a pattern of eating. It's a way of scheduling your meals so that you get the most out of them. Intermittent fasting doesn't change what you eat, it changes when you eat.

Why is it worthwhile to change when you're eating?

Well, most notably, it's a great way to get lean without going on a crazy diet or cutting your calories down to nothing. In fact, most of the time you'll try to keep your calories the same when you start intermittent fasting. (Most people eat bigger meals during a shorter time frame.) Additionally, intermittent fasting is a good way to keep muscle mass on while getting lean.

With all that said, the main reason people try intermittent fasting is to lose fat. We'll talk about how intermittent fasting leads to fat loss in a moment.

Perhaps most importantly, intermittent fasting is one of the simplest strategies we have for taking bad weight off while keeping good weight on because it requires very little behavior change. This is a very good thing because it means intermittent fasting falls into the category of "simple enough that you'll actually do it, but meaningful enough that it will actually make a difference."

How Does Intermittent Fasting Work?

To understand how intermittent fasting leads to fat loss we first need to understand the difference between the fed state and the fasted state.

Your body is in the fed state when it is digesting and absorbing food. Typically, the fed state starts when you begin eating and lasts for three to five hours as your body digests and absorbs the food you just ate. When you are in the fed state, it's very hard for your body to burn fat because your insulin levels are high.

After that timespan, your body goes into what is known as the post–absorptive state, which is just a fancy way of saying that your body isn't processing a meal. The post–absorptive state lasts until 8 to 12 hours after your last meal, which is when you enter the fasted state. It is much easier for you body to burn fat in the fasted state because your insulin levels are low.

When you're in the fasted state your body can burn fat that has been inaccessible during the fed state.

Because we don't enter the fasted state until 12 hours after our last meal, it's rare that our bodies are in this fat burning state. This is one of the reasons why many people who start intermittent fasting will lose fat without changing what they eat, how much they eat, or how often they exercise. Fasting puts your body in a fat burning state that you rarely make it to during a normal eating schedule.

CHAPTER TWO

Techniques of intermittent fasting

Intermittent fasting methods

There are many different ways of intermittent fasting. The methods vary in the number of fast days and the calorie allowances.

Intermittent fasting involves entirely or partially abstaining from eating for a set amount of time, before eating regularly again.

Some studies suggest that this way of eating may offer benefits such as fat loss, better health, and increased longevity. Proponents claim that an intermittent fasting program is easier to maintain than traditional, calorie-controlled diets.

Each person's experience of intermittent fasting is individual, and different styles will suit different people.

In this article, we discuss the research behind the most popular types of intermittent fasting and provide tips on how to maintain this type of diet.

There are various methods of intermittent fasting, and people will prefer different styles. Read on to find out about seven different ways to do intermittent fasting.

1. Fast for 12 hours a day

Different styles of intermittent fasting may suit different people.

The rules for this diet are simple. A person needs to decide on and adhere to a 12-hour fasting window every day.

According to some researchers, fasting for 10–16 hours can cause the body to turn its fat stores into energy, which releases ketones into the bloodstream. This should encourage weight loss.

This type of intermittent fasting plan may be a good option for beginners. This is because the fasting window is relatively small, much of the fasting occurs during sleep, and the person can consume the same number of calories each day.

The easiest way to do the 12-hour fast is to include the period of sleep in the fasting window.

For example, a person could choose to fast between 7 p.m. and 7 a.m. They would need to finish their dinner before 7 p.m. and wait until 7 a.m. to eat breakfast but would be asleep for much of the time in between.

2. Fasting for 16 hours

Fasting for 16 hours a day, leaving an eating window of 8 hours, is called the 16:8 method or the Leangains diet.

During the 16:8 diet, men fast for 16 hours each day, and women fast for 14 hours. This type of intermittent fast may be helpful for someone who has already tried the 12-hour fast but did not see any benefits.

On this fast, people usually finish their evening meal by 8 p.m. and then skip breakfast the next day, not eating again until noon.

A study on mice found that limiting the feeding window to 8 hours protected them from obesity, inflammation, diabetes, and liver disease, even when they ate the same total number of calories as mice that ate whenever they wished.

3. Fasting for 2 days a week

People following the 5:2 diet eat standard amounts of healthful food for 5 days and reduce calorie intake on the other 2 days.

During the 2 fasting days, men generally consume 600 calories and women 500 calories.

Typically, people separate their fasting days in the week. For example, they may fast on a Monday and Thursday and eat normally on the other days. There should be at least 1 non-fasting day between fasting days.

There is limited research on the 5:2 diet, which is also known as the Fast diet. A study involving 107 overweight or obese women found that restricting calories twice weekly and continuous calorie restriction both led to similar weight loss.

The study also found that this diet reduced insulin levels and improved insulin sensitivity among participants.

A small-scale study looked at the effects of this fasting style in 23 overweight women. Over the course of one menstrual cycle, the women lost 4.8 percent of their body weight and 8.0 percent of their total body fat. However, these measurements returned to normal for most of the women after 5 days of normal eating.

4. Alternate day fasting

There are several variations of the alternate day fasting plan, which involves fasting every other day.

For some people, alternate day fasting means a complete avoidance of solid foods on fasting days, while other people allow up to 500 calories. On feeding days, people often choose to eat as much as they want.

One study reports that alternate day fasting is effective for weight loss and heart health in both healthy and overweight adults. The researchers found that the 32 participants lost an average of 5.2 kilograms (kg), or just over 11 pounds (lb), over a 12-week period.

Alternate day fasting is quite an extreme form of intermittent fasting, and it may not be suitable for beginners or those with certain medical conditions. It may also be difficult to maintain this type of fasting in the long term.

5. A weekly 24-hour fast

On a 24-hour diet, a person can have teas and calorie-free drinks.

Fasting completely for 1 or 2 days a week, known as the Eat-Stop-Eat diet, involves eating no food for 24 hours at a time. Many people fast from breakfast to breakfast or lunch to lunch.

People on this diet plan can have water, tea, and other calorie-free drinks during the fasting period.

People should return to normal eating patterns on the non-fasting days. Eating in this manner reduces a person's total calorie intake but does not limit the specific foods that the individual consumes.

A 24-hour fast can be challenging, and it may cause fatigue, headaches, or irritability. Many people find that these effects become less extreme over time as the body adjusts to this new pattern of eating. People may benefit from trying a 12-hour or 16-hour fast before transitioning to the 24-hour fast.

6. Meal skipping

This flexible approach to intermittent fasting may be good for beginners. It involves occasionally skipping meals. People can decide which meals to skip according to their level of hunger or time restraints. However, it is important to eat healthful foods at each meal. Meal skipping is likely to be most successful when individuals monitor and respond to their body's hunger signals. Essentially, people using this style of intermittent fasting will eat when they are hungry and skip meals when they are not.

This may feel more natural for some people than the other fasting methods.

7. The Warrior Diet

The Warrior Diet is a relatively extreme form of intermittent fasting.

The Warrior Diet involves eating very little, usually just a few servings of raw fruit and vegetables, during a 20-hour fasting window, then eating one large meal at night. The eating window is usually only around 4 hours.

This form of fasting may be best for people who have tried other forms of intermittent fasting already. Supporters of the Warrior Diet claim that humans are natural nocturnal eaters and that eating at night allows the body to gain nutrients in line with its circadian rhythms.

During the 4-hour eating phase, people should make sure that they consume plenty of vegetables, proteins, and healthful fats. They should also include some carbohydrates. Although it is possible to eat some foods during the fasting period, it can be challenging to stick to the strict guidelines on when and what to eat in the long term. Also, some people struggle with eating such a large meal so close to bedtime.

There is also a risk that people on this diet will not eat enough nutrients, such as fiber. This can increase the risk of cancer and have an adverse effect on digestive and immune health.

Method 16/8

16:8 intermittent fasting, which people sometimes call the 16:8 diet or 16:8 plan, is a popular type of fasting. People who follow this eating plan will fast for 16 hours a day and consume all of their calories during the remaining 8 hours.

Suggested benefits of the 16:8 plan include weight loss and fat loss, as well as the prevention of type 2 diabetes and other obesity-associated conditions.

Read on to learn more about the 16:8 intermittent fasting plan, including how to do it and the health benefits and side effects.

What is 16:8 intermittent fasting?

Most people on a 16:8 intermittent fasting plan choose to consume their daily calories during the middle part of the day.

16:8 intermittent fasting is a form of time-restricted fasting. It involves consuming foods during an 8-hour window and avoiding food, or fasting, for the remaining 16 hours each day.

Some people believe that this method works by supporting the body's circadian rhythm, which is its internal clock.

Most people who follow the 16:8 plan abstain from food at night and for part of the morning and evening. They tend to consume their daily calories during the middle of the day.

There are no restrictions on the types or amounts of food that a person can eat during the 8-hour window. This flexibility makes the plan relatively easy to follow.

METHOD 5:2

Intermittent fasting is an eating pattern that involves regular fasting.

The 5:2 diet, also known as The Fast Diet, is currently the most popular intermittent fasting diet.

It was popularized by British journalist Michael Mosley.

What is the 5:2 diet?

Eat what you want five days a week, dramatically cut the calories for two. The part-time diet that still allows you to eat chocolate cake yet lose weight has hit the headlines and taken off in a big way.

The practice of fasting has been around for years, with tests carried out to uncover the potential effects as early as the 1940s. However, the dawn of 2013 ushered in a new spin on a practice that had more commonly been associated with religious rituals or even political protests. The intermittent fast, a weight loss wonder (with some other potential but as yet unproven health benefits) was snapped up by the UK dieting community who, feeling the bulge after Christmas 2012, were told they could eat what they wanted for the majority of the week and still lose weight.

The fasting for weight loss phenomenon was actually set in motion in August 2012, when the BBC broadcast a Horizon episode called 'Eat Fast and Live Longer'. Doctor and journalist Michael Mosley presented the diet du jour as 'genuinely revolutionary'; and as a result, published The Fast Diet book in January 2013.

A month after Mosley's book was published, former BBC journalist, Kate Harrison released her version titled The 5:2 Diet Book. The recommendations in both books vary slightly, though the general principles of the diet remain the same.

The diet

The simplicity of the diet, and the fact you can eat pretty much what you like five days a week, are key to its popularity. Dieters are recommended to consume a 'normal' number of calories five days a week and then, for two, non-consecutive days, eat just 25% of their usual calorie total – 500 calories for women and 600 for men.

There are no restrictions on the types of food you can eat and it is suggested that women can expect to lose about 1lb a week on the diet, with men losing about the same if not a little more.

It's called the 5:2 diet because five days of the week are normal eating days, while the other two restrict calories to 500–600 per day.

Because there are no requirements about which foods to eat but rather when you should eat them, this diet is more of a lifestyle.

Many people find this way of eating to be easier to stick to than a traditional calorie-restricted diet (1Trusted Source).

How to Do the 5:2 Diet

The 5:2 diet is actually very simple to explain.

For five days per week, you eat normally and don't have to think about restricting calories.

Then, on the other two days, you reduce your calorie intake to a quarter of your daily needs. This is about 500 calories per day for women, and 600 for men.

You can choose whichever two days of the week you prefer, as long as there is at least one non-fasting day in between them.

One common way of planning the week is to fast on Mondays and Thursdays, with two or three small meals, then eat normally for the rest of the week.

It's important to emphasize that eating "normally" does not mean you can eat anything. If you binge on junk food, then you probably won't lose any weight, and you may even gain weight.

You should eat the same amount of food as if you hadn't been fasting at all.

There are very few studies on the 5:2 diet specifically.

However, there are plenty of studies on intermittent fasting in general, which show impressive health benefits.

One important benefit is that intermittent fasting seems to be easier to follow than continuous calorie restriction, at least for some people.

Also, many studies have shown that different types of intermittent fasting may significantly reduce insulin levels.

One study showed that the 5:2 diet caused weight loss similar to regular calorie restriction. Additionally, the diet was very effective at reducing insulin levels and improving insulin sensitivity.

Several studies have looked into the health effects of modified alternate-day fasting, which is very similar to the 5:2 diet (ultimately, it's a 4:3 diet).

The 4:3 diet may help reduce insulin resistance, asthma, seasonal allergies, heart arrhythmias, menopausal hot flashes and more.

One randomized controlled study in both normal-weight and overweight individuals showed major improvements in the group doing 4:3 fasting, compared to the control group that ate normally.

After 12 weeks, the fasting group had:

Reduced body weight by more than 11 pounds (5 kg).

Reduced fat mass by 7.7 pounds (3.5 kg), with no change in muscle mass.

Reduced blood levels of triglycerides by 20%.

Increased LDL particle size, which is a good thing.

Reduced levels of CRP, an important marker of inflammation.

Decreased levels of leptin by up to 40%.

The 5:2 Diet for Weight Loss

If you need to lose weight, the 5:2 diet can be very effective when done right.

This is mainly because the 5:2 eating pattern helps you consume fewer calories.

Therefore, it is very important not to compensate for the fasting days by eating much more on the non-fasting days.

Intermittent fasting does not cause more weight loss than regular calorie restriction if total calories are matched.

That said, fasting protocols similar to the 5:2 diet have shown a lot of promise in weight loss studies:

A recent review found that modified alternate-day fasting led to weight loss of 3–8% over the course of 3–24 weeks (15).

In the same study, participants lost 4–7% of their waist circumference, meaning that they lost a lot of harmful belly fat.

Intermittent fasting causes a much smaller reduction in muscle mass when compared to weight loss with conventional calorie restriction.

Intermittent fasting is even more effective when combined with exercise, such as endurance or strength training.

How to Eat on Fasting Days

There is no rule for what or when to eat on fasting days.

Some people function best by beginning the day with a small breakfast, while others find it best to start eating as late as possible.

Generally, there are two meal patterns that people follow:

1. **Three small meals: Usually breakfast, lunch and dinner.**
2. **Two slightly bigger meals: Only lunch and dinner.**

Since calorie intake is limited — 500 calories for women and 600 calories for men — it makes sense to use your calorie budget wisely.

Try to focus on nutritious, high-fiber, high-protein foods that will make you feel full without consuming too many calories.

Soups are a great option on fast days. Studies have shown that they may make you feel more full than the same ingredients in original form, or foods with the same calorie content.

Here are a few examples of foods that may be suitable for fast days:

1. *A generous portion of vegetables*
2. *Natural yogurt with berries*
3. *Boiled or baked eggs.*
4. *Grilled fish or lean meat*
5. *Cauliflower rice*
6. *Soups (for example miso, tomato, cauliflower or vegetable)*
7. *Low-calorie cup soups*
8. *Black coffee*
9. *Tea*
10. *Still or sparkling water*

There is no specific, correct way to eat on fasting days. You have to experiment and figure out what works best for you.

THE WARRIOR DIET

What Is the Warrior Diet?

The warrior diet is a type of intermittent fasting protocol that involves extended periods of fasting and short periods of feasting. The feasting portion of the warrior diet is quite literal — dieters are encouraged to eat 85 to 90 percent of their calories during this window, which can be up to 1,800 calories in one sitting for someone on a typical 2,000 calorie plan or up to 2,700 calories in one sitting for an active person who needs 3,000 calories per day.

"The warrior diet is a stricter type of intermittent fasting, alternating between 20 hours of undereating and 4 hours of unlimited intake. Experts worry this diet may lead to nutrient deficiencies and warn that it is inappropriate for many groups (like athletes or pregnant women)."

Fasting is nothing new, and the practice of fasting has a diverse, complex history. Perhaps the earliest records of fasting go back to ancient Greece when philosopher Pythagoras touted the virtues of fasting. Hippocrates and other prominent healers, like the Renaissance doctor Paracelsus, were also advocates of fasting.   Fasting has been a critical component of nearly all the world's major religions — Judaism recognizes multiple fasting days throughout the year; Muslims fast during the holy month of Ramadan, and Christians observe a 40-day fast during Lent.

Fasting has also been used as a means for political protest, as evidenced by the Suffragette hunger strikes and Mahatma Gandhi's fasting episodes during the struggle for Indian independence.

Now, fasting is a popular weight-loss or performance-enhancement protocol in the wellness world. Intermittent fasting, in particular, has skyrocketed in popularity because of its profound effects on weight loss and body composition. The science community has also endorsed intermittent fasting for its health benefits on the heart, brain, and other organs.

The warrior diet is a type of intermittent fasting developed by Ori Hofmekler, a renowned author in the world of health and fitness. Hofmekler created the diet in 2001 after years of observing himself and his colleagues in the Israeli Special Forces.

It's important to note that the warrior diet isn't based on science in the clinical sense — instead, the warrior diet is based on Hofmekler's own observations and opinions on the tactics he used to stay fit during his time in the military.

How It Works

The warrior diet involves fasting for 20 hours overnight and during the day, and then overeating during a four-hour window in the evening. This principle is based on the idea that our primitive ancestors spent their days hunting and gathering and would feast at night.

What Is Intermittent Fasting?

What To Eat

Technically, there aren't any off-limits foods on the warrior diet. It's encouraged that you consume nutrient-dense foods and get in plenty of fruits, vegetables, and protein, but you could just as easily reach for a pizza during your four-hour eating window.

Hofmekler suggests that your meals should be based around healthy fats and large portions of protein, specifically dairy protein sources such as cheese and yogurt. There's no need to count calories on the warrior diet if you follow Hofmekler's suggestions and focus on unprocessed foods.

Compliant Foods

- *Fruit and Vegetables: Try to consume a few servings of fruits and vegetables each day in order to ensure you get enough essential vitamins and minerals.*

- *Grains: Whole grain foods, such as sprouted wheat bread, quinoa, rice, bulgur and oatmeal are all great options to fuel up on during your eating window.*
- *Dairy: The warrior diet particularly encourages dairy foods, especially raw and full-fat ones. Hofmekler is a fan of cheese, yogurt, and raw milk.*
- *Protein: People on the warrior diet are urged to consume large amounts of protein. Protein is essential for maintaining and building muscle mass, a key goal outcome of the warrior diet.*
- *Beverages: On the warrior diet, you can consume any zero-calorie beverages during your fasting window, and essentially anything you want during your feeding window. The diet recommends water, black coffee, and milk.*

Non-compliant Foods

Again, there aren't any foods that are totally off-limits for the warrior diet, but there are some foods you should try to keep to a minimum on any diet:

1. *Sugary Processed Foods: Packaged sugary foods are one of the main culprits behind many chronic diseases, including diabetes and inflammatory bowel disorders. Try to keep added sugar to a minimum.*

2. *Salty Processed Foods: Even though they might seem healthier than sugary foods, salty snacks can be just as damaging to your blood sugar and other health markers. If you're looking for something crunchy and savory, try veggies with hummus or guacamole. You can also make your own savory snacks at home.*

3. *Sugary Beverages: Try to keep your intake of soda, energy drinks and juice with added sugars low. Sugary beverages are a leading cause of weight gain, tooth decay, and illness.*

Recommended Timing

Timing is the key component of the warrior diet. The entire protocol is based around the idea that long periods of fasting and short windows of overeating lead to optimal health, fitness, and body composition.

During the 20-hour fasting period, you should consume only minimal calories. Hofmekler encourages dieters to sustain themselves on small portions of dairy, hard-boiled eggs, and raw produce. You can also drink zero-calorie beverages, including coffee, during the fasting period.

When it's time for your feeding window, you can essentially eat however much of whatever you want until the four hours are over. You can determine your feeding window based on a timeframe that works well for you, but most people save their feast for the evening hours.

When it's time for your feeding window, you can essentially eat however much of whatever you want until the four hours are over. You can determine your feeding window based on a timeframe that works well for you, but most people save their feast for the evening hours.

Modifications

There aren't any modifications to the warrior diet itself. If you deviate off of the 20:4 protocol, you wouldn't be on the warrior diet anymore. However, there are many other intermittent fasting protocols that may be more beneficial and have more research behind them.

Those include the 16:8 method, the 5:2 diet, Eat-Stop-Eat, and alternate-day fasting. See the Similar Diets section for more intermittent fasting protocols.

Pros and Cons

Pros

1. May aid weight loss

2. May improve blood sugar

3. May help with inflammation

4. May reduce risk of cognitive disease

Cons

1. Difficult to follow

2. May lead to binge eating

3. Inappropriate for many groups

4. Many potential side effects

5. Nutrient deficiencies

Pros

1. **May Aid Weight Loss:** There's a great deal of evidence that links intermittent fasting to weight loss, including 20-hour cycles. Consistent alternate-day fasting has been shown to help overweight people lose a substantial amount of body fat and decrease the risk of cardiovascular disease.

2. **May Improve Blood Sugar:** Fasting is strongly associated with improvements in blood sugar control and insulin sensitivity. This potential benefit can be lost, however, if you choose to eat high-carbohydrate or sugary foods during your feeding window.

3. **May Help With Inflammation:** Inflammation is a leading cause of disease, including heart disease, diabetes, some cancers, bowel disorders and more. Research suggests that intermittent fasting could be a good way to combat chronic inflammation.

4. **May Reduce Risk of Cognitive Disease**: Animal studies have found that intermittent fasting may have a protective effect against cognitive decline and diseases such as Alzheimer's disease. The research in this area is fledgling, however, and more studies are needed to confirm this effect.

Cons

1. **Difficult to Follow:** While our paleolithic ancestors may have easily gone 20 hours without food, that's not a norm in modern society and we aren't conditioned to follow that pattern. Fasting for 20 hours every day is very difficult, and you may experience severe cravings, hunger and other symptoms.

2. **May Lead to Binge Eating:** Although reduced calorie intake is common in many fasting protocols, it's possible that you could consume too many calories during your four-hour on the warrior diet window due to cravings or feelings of deprivation. You may also experience obsessive thoughts about food during the fasting period.

3. **Inappropriate for Many Groups:** Many people should not follow the warrior diet, including women who are pregnant or nursing.

4. **Many Potential Side Effects:** Depriving your body of substantial calories can lead to fatigue, brain fog or difficulty focusing, "hanger", mood swings, stress, anxiety, dizziness or lightheadedness, hormonal disruptions and more.

5. **Nutrient Deficiencies:** Because your eating is restricted to so few hours, it may be difficult to consume the recommended servings of fruits and vegetables,

especially when you may be focused on more carb-heavy or protein-dense foods.

How It Compares

USDA Recommendations

The federal dietary recommendations include five food groups: fruit, vegetables, grains, dairy, and protein.

The key recommendations in the federal guidelines include:

A variety of vegetables from all of the subgroups—dark green, red and orange, legumes (beans and peas), starchy, and other

Fruits, especially whole fruits

Grains, at least half of which are whole grains

Fat-free or low-fat dairy, including milk, yogurt, cheese, and/or fortified soy beverages

A variety of protein foods, including seafood, lean meats and poultry, eggs, legumes (beans and peas), and nuts, seeds, and soy products

Oils

Limited saturated fats, trans fats, added sugars and sodium"

The warrior diet encourages dieters to eat raw fruits and vegetables, dairy, whole grains and protein, so on the surface, it seems this diet is consistent with the federal recommendation. However, dieters are really free to choose whatever foods they want, so there's no guarantee that you will consume enough nutrients on the warrior diet. Additionally, it's hard to consume the recommended amount of nutrient-dense foods in just four hours.

CHAPTER THREE

The 16/8 method4 step by step

The easiest way to follow the 16:8 diet is to choose a 16-hour fasting window that includes the time that a person spends sleeping.

Some experts advise finishing food consumption in the early evening, as metabolism slows down after this time. However, this is not feasible for everyone.

Some people may not be able to consume their evening meal until 7 p.m. or later. Even so, it is best to avoid food for 2–3 hours before bed.

People may choose one of the following 8-hour eating windows:

1. 9 a.m. to 5 p.m.
2. 10 a.m. to 6 p.m.
3. noon to 8 p.m.

Within this timeframe, people can eat their meals and snacks at convenient times. Eating regularly is important to prevent blood sugar peaks and dips and to avoid excessive hunger.

Some people may need to experiment to find the best eating window and mealtimes for their lifestyle.

Recommended foods and tips

While the 16:8 intermittent fasting plan does not specify which foods to eat and avoid, it is beneficial to focus on healthful eating and to limit or avoid junk foods. The consumption of too much unhealthful food may cause weight gain and contribute to disease.

A balanced diet focuses primarily on:

fruits and vegetables, which can be fresh, frozen, or canned (in water)

whole grains, including quinoa, brown rice, oats, and barley

lean protein sources, such as poultry, fish, beans, lentils, tofu, nuts, seeds, low fat cottage cheese, and eggs

healthful fats from fatty fish, olives, olive oil, coconuts, avocados, nuts, and seeds

Fruits, vegetables, and whole grains are high in fiber, so they can help keep a person feeling full and satisfied. Healthful fats and proteins can also contribute to satiety.

Beverages can play a role in satiety for those following the 16:8 intermittent fasting diet. Drinking water regularly throughout the day can help reduce calorie intake because people often mistake thirst for hunger.

The 16:8 diet plan permits the consumption of calorie-free drinks — such as water and unsweetened tea and coffee — during the 16-hour fasting window. It is important to consume fluids regularly to avoid dehydration.

Tips

- People may find it easier to stick to the 16:8 diet when they follow these tips:
- drinking cinnamon herbal tea during the fasting period, as it may suppress the appetite
- consuming water regularly throughout the day
- watching less television to reduce exposure to images of food, which may stimulate a sense of hunger
- exercising just before or during the eating window, as exercise can trigger hunger
- practicing mindful eating when consuming meals
- trying meditation during the fasting period to allow hunger pangs to pass

Health benefits

Researchers have been studying intermittent fasting for decades.

Study findings are sometimes contradictory and inconclusive. However, the research on intermittent fasting, including 16:8 fasting, indicates that it may provide the following benefits:

Weight loss and fat loss

Eating during a set period can help people reduce the number of calories that they consume. It may also help boost metabolism.

A 2017 study suggests that intermittent fasting leads to greater weight loss and fat loss in men with obesity than regular calorie restriction.

Research from 2016 reports that men who followed a 16:8 approach for 8 weeks while resistance training showed a decrease in fat mass. The participants maintained their muscle mass throughout.

In contrast, a 2017 study found very little difference in weight loss between participants who practiced intermittent fasting — in the form of alternate-day fasting rather than 16:8 fasting — and those who reduced their overall calorie intake. The dropout rate was also high among those in the intermittent fasting group.

Disease prevention

Supporters of intermittent fasting suggest that it can prevent several conditions and diseases, including:

- **type 2 diabetes**
- **heart conditions**
- **some cancers**
- **neurodegenerative diseases**

A 2014 review reports that intermittent fasting shows promise as an alternative to traditional calorie restriction for type 2 diabetes risk reduction and weight loss in people who have overweight or obesity.

The researchers caution, however, that more research is necessary before they can reach reliable conclusions.

A 2018 study indicates that in addition to weight loss, an 8-hour eating window may help reduce blood pressure in adults with obesity.

Other studies report that intermittent fasting reduces fasting glucose by 3–6% in those with prediabetes, although it has no effect on healthy individuals. It may also decrease fasting insulin by 11–57% after 3 to 24 weeks of intermittent fasting.

Time-restricted fasting, such as the 16:8 method, may also protect learning and memory and slow down diseases that affect the brain.

A 2017 annual review notes that animal research has indicated that this form of fasting reduces the risk of nonalcoholic fatty liver disease and cancer.

Extended life span

Animal studies suggest that intermittent fasting may help animals live longer. For example, one study found that short-term repeated fasting increased the life span of female mice.

The National Institute on Aging point out that, even after decades of research, scientists still cannot explain why fasting may lengthen life span. As a result, they cannot confirm the long-term safety of this practice.

Human studies in the area are limited, and the potential benefits of intermittent fasting for human longevity are not yet known.

Side effects and risks

16:8 intermittent fasting has some associated risks and side effects. As a result, the plan is not right for everyone.

Potential side effects and risks include:

- hunger, weakness, and tiredness in the beginning stages of the plan
- overeating or eating unhealthful foods during the 8-hour eating window due to excessive hunger
- heartburn or reflux as a result of overeating

Intermittent fasting may be less beneficial for women than men. Some research on animals suggests that intermittent fasting could negatively affect female fertility.

Individuals with a history of disordered eating may wish to avoid intermittent fasting. The National Eating Disorders Association warn that fasting is a risk factor for eating disorders.

The 16:8 plan may also not be suitable for those with a history of depression and anxiety. Some research indicates that short-term calorie restriction might relieve depression but that chronic calorie restriction can have the opposite effect. More research is necessary to understand the implications of these findings.

16:8 intermittent fasting is unsuitable for those who are pregnant, breastfeeding, or trying to conceive.

The National Institute on Aging conclude that there is insufficient evidence to recommend any fasting diet, especially for older adults.

People who wish to try the 16:8 method or other types of intermittent fasting should talk to their doctor first, especially if they are taking medications or have:

- an underlying health condition, such as diabetes or low blood pressure
- a history of disordered eating
- a history of mental health disorders

Anyone who has any concerns or experiences any adverse effects of the diet should see a doctor.

Diabetes

While evidence indicates that the 16:8 method may be helpful for diabetes prevention, it may not be suitable for those who already have the condition.

The 16:8 intermittent fasting diet is not suitable for people with type 1 diabetes. However, some people with prediabetes or type 2 diabetes may be able to try the diet under a doctor's supervision.

People with diabetes who wish to try the 16:8 intermittent fasting plan should see their doctor before making changes to their eating habits.

CHAPTER FOUR

POTENTIALS OF "IF"

Why the Potential Intermittent Fasting Benefits Might Not Be Worth the Risks

Any dietitian or nutritionist will likely admit that they have a list of the questions most commonly asked by clients. Typically, that list evolves based on the latest diet and wellness trends—a couple of years ago, everyone wanted to talk about the paleo diet, and while the Whole30 craze is still alive and well, I get a lot more questions now about the keto diet. Another big one right now: intermittent fasting.

What is intermittent fasting?

More of an "eating pattern" than an actual diet, intermittent fasting (IF) is characterized by cycling between periods of eating and fasting. There are several approaches, but the most popular are those that involve either daily 16-hour fasts in which you eat all your food in an eight-hour window, or an IF pattern in which someone fasts for 24 hours, usually twice per week. There's also the 5:2 plan, where you eat "normally" for five days and then for the other two days, consume only about 500 to 600 calories.

While there are exceptions, in general, IF patterns tell you when to eat, but not necessarily what to eat.

What are the intermittent fasting benefits?

While research has shown some potential health benefits of intermittent fasting, as a dietitian and health coach who focuses on sustainable lifestyle approaches to wellness, I can't quite get on board with recommending that someone just not eat. Fasting can be a slippery slope to unhealthy habits and a screwy relationship with food.

That doesn't mean I won't work with someone who wants to explore IF-it just means we need to discuss why you're interested in using this method to reach your goals and whether there might be other options to achieve the health benefits you're after in a more sustainable way.

Weight management is probably the number-one reason people ask me about intermittent fasting. While studies have shown that intermittent fasting benefits may include weight loss and improved metabolism, this eating pattern has also been researched for its impact on insulin resistance, as well as for its potential to decrease inflammation, enhance cell repair, and support a healthy gastrointestinal tract. Sounds great, right? Not so fast.

Here are the health concerns about intermittent fasting.

The main issue that comes up is sustainability—meaning, can you maintain this way of eating, and, more so, should you? Many people find they feel great while following an intermittent fasting plan but struggle when they try to stick with it for a prolonged period. Figuring out how to fit those fasting and eating periods into your work and social life, and fuel and refuel appropriately around your workouts, can be a logistical nightmare and also a health challenge. This is especially true if you work long days, wake up really early, or go to bed very late. It can also be tricky for people who lack a sense of routine in their day-to-day life. While some people have found it motivates them to get into a more consistent schedule, many have gotten frustrated for not being able to keep it up. When your self-esteem takes a hit like that, it can trickle into other areas of your life.

I've seen many people who hop on and off the IF bandwagon start to feel out of touch with their hunger and fullness cues. This mind-body disconnect can make it difficult to establish an overall healthy diet for the long haul. For certain people, this could lead to or resurface disordered eating behaviors. (BTW, have you heard of orthorexia? It's the eating disorder masking itself as a healthy diet.)

If you still want to try intermittent fasting...

With all that said, if you've consulted your doctor and/or your certified nutritionist, and you're intrigued by the potential benefits of intermittent fasting, here are a few tips to keep in mind.

Identify what intermittent fasting benefits you after.

Are you hoping to lose weight with intermittent fasting? Is there another health reason? Have you tried other approaches to meeting your goal? If yes, why didn't they work? Zeroing in on what intermittent fasting health effects you hope to accomplish and the motivations behind them will help you prioritize foods and strategies that help you get there in a healthy way.

Consider your approach.

Decide whether a daily 16/8 approach or something more like a weekly 5:2 plan will work better for your stomach and schedule. When do you usually get hungry throughout the day? What time do you wake up and go to bed? How often and what time of the day do you work out? All of this will help determine when you are in fasting mode. For example, if you routinely hit the sack after midnight, closing the kitchen at 6 p.m. probably won't be so easy.

Make intermittent fasting work around you.

Take into account when you tend to go to sleep and wake up. Then factor in when you like to exercise. What is your work schedule like? How about your social life? This will help you figure out how to spread out your fasting and eating phases, so you're never starving, cranky, and struggling to maintain your energy and focus.

Have an exit strategy.

Are you thinking of IF as a long-term plan? While I don't recommend it as such, if you intend to be intermittently fasting forever (whew), you better make sure you have a plan to help reintroduce a more regular eating schedule back into your life. I see a lot of people trip up when they try to come off an IF cycle because they can't seem to get reacquainted with their appetite and hunger cues. If you're serious about doing IF in a healthy, mindful way, come up with a post-IF plan (perhaps together with a dietitian) so you have something to guide you.

GETTING THE MOST OUT OF EXERCISE

Lastly, after applying all of these tips, do yourself a favor and exercise. There's no need to enroll in a gym membership, there are plenty of workouts that can be done in the comfort of your home. They'll boost your energy, improve your muscle strength and endurance, and help your body burn fat fast.

INTERMITTENT FASTING HACKS

Another diet plan that's rapidly growing in popularity now is intermittent fasting. It's a diet concept where you fast for a set period of time during the day—usually between 14-18 consecutive hours—and eat during the other 4-8 hours of the day, while focusing on eating healthy and nutritious food. It's proven to help lose weight, prevent certain diseases, and improve your overall health.

And to help you get started on your intermittent fasting journey, here are some great tips and tricks that'll help you stick to weight loss goals. These are ideas that are all easy to implement, have impressive results, and will make your diet plan easier. So check them out and let me know what you think!

After fasting for 16 hours, don't let yourself think that you can now eat anything you want. Rather, focus on eating whole foods that'll fill up your body with the essentials vitamins and nutrition you need. This will boost your energy and balance your hormones throughout the whole fasting period.

Avoid Artificially Flavored Drinks

Ditch the diet soda, energy drinks, and other flavored beverages that say they're low in sugar. They actually have a lot of artificial sweeteners that are horrible for your health. They use things like

Splenda or Sweet & Low which stimulate your appetite and cause you to overeat.

Drink More Water

One of the most important factors in any diet plan is to make sure your body is well hydrated. By simply drinking a glass of water before each meal, the water will suppress your appetite and make you feel fuller sooner (so you can avoid overeating).

Also, try adding some fresh fruit and herbs to your water for a detoxifying drink. It's tasty and totally healthy.

Keep Yourself Busy During the Fasting Hours

Whenever possible, during the fasting hours, make sure you're being busy and productive. Try taking a walk in the park, write in your journal, run some errands, or read your favorite book. These are just simple tricks that'll distract you from thinking about food.

Get Enough Sleep

Sleep is a vital indicator of your overall health and well-being. It helps repair your body and lose weight. And the reason for this is because our bodies burn calories while performing certain functions while sleeping and which also boosts your metabolism.

Control Your Stress

Stress can trigger overeating which makes intermittent fasting seem nearly impossible to maintain. When you're influenced by stress and lack of good sleep, you'll tend to focus on eating unhealthy food to make yourself feel better. So learn to control your stress while on this diet.

Remember Fasting Means Zero

While on the intermittent fasting diet, always be true to yourself and disciplined. By simply not eating any food during the fasting hours, this will help you make sure you're losing weight at the speed you want.

CHAPTER SIX

INTERMITTENT FASTING AND THE KETOGENIC DIET

What is the Keto Diet:

Put simply; the ketogenic diet is a diet that is high in fat and very low in carbs which forces your body to start a process called nutritional ketosis. This means your body starts to burn stored fats for energy due to the lack of glucose in the bloodstream.

Glucose, also known as the body's primary fuel source, is converted from carbohydrates. This is found in dozens of everyday food items — from white bread to fruits and vegetables.

Limiting these carb-rich foods to 25g a day is paramount to the ketogenic diet, but it doesn't stop there.

To supply your body's nutritional needs while maintaining ketosis, you will actually shift to eating high-fat foods with a moderate amount of protein. For example Fish, certain nuts, eggs, and most meat sources.

As far as benefits go, the keto diet is usually applied with weight loss in mind. However, it is also shown to result in a number of benefits including increased energy levels, healthier inflammatory response, and improved blood sugar balance (among other things).

Combining the Keto Diet with Intermittent Fasting

By understanding their individual uses, you may think that the Keto diet and IF will be too taxing on the body when used together.

However, Based on research, I believe that I have found the perfect way to piece them together into a single system and with the right implementation, one can incorporate the effects of being in ketosis with that of fasting.

For example, while gaining muscle mass is much harder with a ketogenic diet, IF solves this by improving the body's insulin sensitivity, blood glucose regulation, and growth hormone production.

Fasting can also help your body achieve ketosis much faster.

Once you are in ketosis, it will be much easier to stick to your IF schedule since you will experience fewer hunger pains.

Remember that IF keeps your metabolism high, which helps you adapt quickly to your reduced carb intake.

Finally, being in ketosis while fasting allows your body to start using your body fat as a fuel source which leads to lower BF% and a leaner body overall.

If all these are proven to be true, then the Keto and IF combination would be a breakthrough.

Snacks? No Snacks!

No snacking! Well, you can snack, but try to stay away from it as much as you can. You want your body to stay in a fasting state until the beginning of your eating window. If you're snacking, then you will interrupt the process.

CHAPTER SEVEN

30 day intermittent fasting meal plan

WEEK1

MONDAY

Breakfast

YUMMY BIG AVOCADO BALLS

Lunch:

ULTIMATE KETO COFFEE CAKE

Dinner:

PARMESAN GARLIC BREAD RECIPE

TUESDAY

Breakfast:

KETO GREEN FINGERS SALAD

Lunch:

LOW CARB KEY LIME CHEESECAKES

Dinner:

GINGER SOY BOK CHOY RECIPE

WEDNESDAY

Breakfast:

CHEESE STUFFED BACON WRAPPED HOT DOGS

Lunch:

CARAMEL POTS DE CRÈM

Dinner:

ASIAN-BRINED PORK CHOPS RECIPE

THURSDAY

Breakfast:

5 MINUTE KETO EGG DROP SOUP

Lunch:

PECAN BUTTER CHIA SEED BLONDIES

Dinner:

GARLIC NOODLES RECIPE

FRIDAY

Breakfast:

RISPY TOFU AND BOK CHOY SALAD

Lunch:

KETO PUMPKIN SNICKERDOODLE COOKIES

Dinner:

CINNAMON ROLL "OATMEAL"

SATURDAY

Breakfast:

KETOGENIC NASI LEMAK

Lunch:

FRIED QUESO FRESCO

Dinner:

ROASTED ASPARAGUS WITH GARLIC RECIPE

SUNDAY

Breakfast:

LOW CARB SAUSAGE AND PEPPER SOUP

Lunch:

RED PEPPER SPINACH SALAD

Dinner:

BAKED CHICKEN AND POTATO CASSEROLE RECIPE

WEEK2

MONDAY

Breakfast:

KETO PIGS IN A BLANKET

Lunch:

BACON INFUSED SUGAR SNAP PEAS

Dinner:

ITALIAN SHRIMP PASTA RECIPE

TUESDAY

Breakfast:

BBQ BACON WRAPPED SMOKIES

Lunch:

BACON JAMMIN' GREEN BEANS

Dinner:

GARLIC PARMESAN ROASTED CARROTS RECIPE

WEDNESDAY

Breakfast:

KETO ROTI JOHN

Lunch:

ROASTED PECAN GREEN BEAN

Dinner:

GARLIC HERB GRILLED SALMON RECIPE

THURSDAY

Breakfast:

ROASTED RED BELL PEPPER AND CAULIFLOWER SOUP

Lunch:

BOK CHOY CHICKEN RECIPE

Dinner:

KETO PUMPKIN SNICKERDOODLE COOKIES

FRIDAY

Breakfast:

SOUTHWESTERN PORK STEW

Lunch:

GARLIC BUTTER STEAK RECIPE

Dinner:

FRIED QUESO FRESCO

SATURDAY

Breakfast:

CHICKEN ENCHILADA SOUP

Lunch:

PARMESAN GARLIC BREAD RECIPE

Dinner:

RED PEPPER SPINACH SALAD

SUNDAY

Breakfast:

THAI PEANUT SHRIMP CURRY

Lunch:

GINGER SOY BOK CHOY RECIPE

Dinner:

BACON INFUSED SUGAR SNAP PEAS

WEEK3

MONDAY

Breakfast:

KETO GRILLED CHEESE SANDWICH

Lunch:

ASIAN-BRINED PORK CHOPS RECIPE

Dinner:

BACON JAMMIN' GREEN BEANS

TUESDAY

Breakfast:

FRESH BELL PEPPER BASIL PIZZA

Lunch:

GARLIC NOODLES RECIPE

Dinner:

ROASTED PECAN GREEN BEAN

Breakfast:

LOW CARB PASTA A LA CARBONARA

Lunch:

CINNAMON ROLL "OATMEAL"

Dinner:

BOK CHOY CHICKEN RECIPE

Breakfast:

SPICY JALAPENO POPPERS

Lunch:

ROASTED ASPARAGUS WITH GARLIC RECIPE

Dinner:

GARLIC BUTTER STEAK RECIPE

Breakfast:

ASIAN CUCUMBER SALAD

Lunch:

BAKED CHICKEN AND POTATO CASSEROLE RECIPE

Dinner:

REVERSE SEARED RIBEYE STEAK

Breakfast:

LOW CARB MOROCCAN MEATBALLS

Lunch:

ITALIAN SHRIMP PASTA RECIPE

Dinner:

KETO TATER TOT NACHOS (AKA TOTCHOS)

Breakfast:

PORTOBELLO PERSONAL PIZZAS

Lunch:

GARLIC PARMESAN ROASTED CARROTS RECIPE

Dinner:

BLACKBERRY CHIPOTLE CHICKEN WING

WEEK4

MONDAY

Breakfast:

KETO THAI CHICKEN FLATBREAD PIZZA

Lunch:

GARLIC HERB GRILLED SALMON RECIPE

Dinner:

KETO CHICKEN PAD THAI

TUESDAY

Breakfast:

REVERSE SEARED RIBEYE STEAK

Lunch:

KETO PIGS IN A BLANKET

Dinner:

LOW-CARB CHICKEN CURRY

WEDNESDAY

Breakfast:

KETO TATER TOT NACHOS (AKA TOTCHOS)

Lunch:

BBQ BACON WRAPPED SMOKIES

Dinner:

THAI CHICKEN ZOODLES

THURSDAY

Breakfast:

BLACKBERRY CHIPOTLE CHICKEN WING

Lunch:

KETO ROTI JOHN

Dinner:

ULTIMATE KETO COFFEE CAKE

Breakfast:

KETO CHICKEN PAD THAI

Lunch:

ROASTED RED BELL PEPPER AND CAULIFLOWER SOUP

Dinner:

LOW CARB KEY LIME CHEESECAKES

Breakfast:

LOW-CARB CHICKEN CURRY

Lunch:

SOUTHWESTERN PORK STEW

Dinner:

CARAMEL POTS DE CRÈM

SUNDAY

Breakfast:

THAI CHICKEN ZOODLES

Lunch:

CHICKEN ENCHILADA SOUP

Dinner:

THAI PEANUT SHRIMP CURRY

YUMMY BIG AVOCADO BALLS

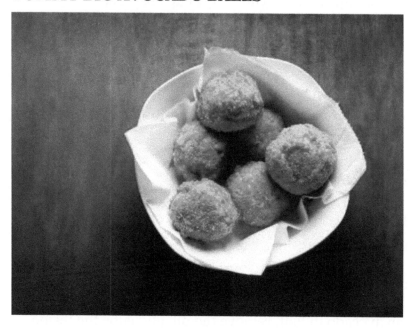

INGREDIENTS

• 10 oz. Canned Tuna, drained

• 1/4 cup Mayonnaise

• 1 medium Avocado, cubed

• 1/4 cup Parmesan Cheese

• 1/3 cup Almond Flour

73

- 1/2 tsp. Garlic Powder

- 1/4 tsp. Onion Powder

- Salt and Pepper to Taste

- 1/2 cup Coconut Oil, for frying (~1/4 cup absorbed)

INSTRUCTION

1. Drain a can of tuna and add it to a large container where you'll be able to

mix everything together.

2. Add mayonnaise, parmesan cheese, and spices to the tuna and mix toge-

ther well.

3. Slice an avocado in half, remove the pit, and cube the inside.

4. Add avocado into the tuna mixture and fold together, trying to not mash the avocado into the mixture.

5. Form the tuna mixture into balls and roll into almond flour, covering completely. Set aside.

6. Heat coconut oil in a pan over medium heat. Once hot, add tuna balls and fry until crisp on all sides.

7. Remove from the pan and serve.

This makes a total of 12 Avocado Tuna Melt Bites.

Per bite, each comes out to be 135 Calories, 11.8g Fats, 0.8g Net Carbs, and 6.2g Protein.

KETO MIXED GREEN SPRING SALAD

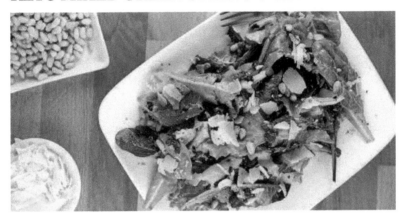

INGREDIENTS

• 2 OZ. Mixed Greens

• 3 tbsp. Pine Nuts, roasted

• 2 tbsp. 5 Minute Keto Raspberry Vinaigrette

• 2 tbsp. Shaved Parmesan

• 2 slices Bacon

• Salt and Pepper to taste

INSTRUCTION

1. Cook bacon until very crisp. You can let it burn slightly on the edges to give the salad a slight addition in bitter notes in some bites.

2. Measure out your greens and set in a container that can be shaken.

3. Crumble bacon, then add the rest of the ingredients to the greens. Shake the container with a lid on to distribute the dressing and contents evenly.

4. Serve and enjoy!

This makes a total of 1 serving of Keto Mixed Green Spring Salad.

The macros come out to be 478 Calories, 37.3g Fats, 4.3g Net Carbs, and 17.1g Protein.

CHEESE STUFFED BACON WRAPPED HOT DOGS

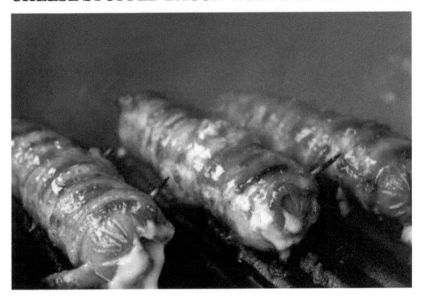

INGREDIENTS

- 6 Hot Dogs

- 12 slices Bacon

- 2 oz. Cheddar Cheese

- 1/2 tsp. Garlic Powder

- 1/2 tsp. Onion Powder

- Salt and Pepper to Taste

INSTRUCTION

1. Pre-heat oven to 400F. Make a slit in all of the hot dogs to make room for the cheese.

2. Slice 2 oz. Cheddar cheese from a block into small long rectangles and stuff into the hot dogs.

3. Start by tightly wrapping one slice of bacon around the hot dog.

4. Continue tightly wrapping the second slice of bacon around the hot dog, slightly overlapping with the first slice.

5. Poke toothpicks through each side of the bacon and hot dog, securing the bacon in place.

6. Set on a wire rack that's on top of a cookie sheet. Season with garlic pow-der, onion powder, salt and pepper.

7. Bake for 35-40 minutes, or until bacon is crispy. Additionally broil the bacon on top if needed.

8. Serve up with some delicious creamed spinach!

This makes a total of 6 Cheese Stuffed Bacon Wrapped Hot Dogs.

Each comes out to be 380 Calories, 34.5g Fats, 0.3g Net Carbs, and 16.8g Protein

5 MINUTE KETO EGG DROP SOUP

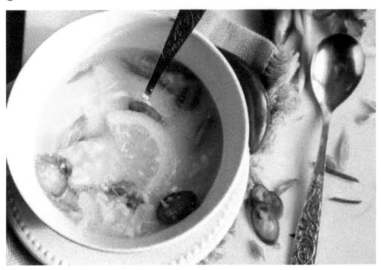

INGREDIENTS

- 1 1/2 cups Chicken Broth

- 1/2 cube Chicken Boullion

- 1 tbsp. Bacon Fat (or butter)

- 2 large Eggs

- 1 tsp. Chili Garlic Paste

INSTRUCTION

1. Put a pan on the stove and turn it to medium-high right away. You want to get this done quick so hotter is better in this circumstance. Add to it the chic-ken broth, boullion cube, and bacon fat (or butter).

2. Bring the broth to a boil and stir everything together. Then, add the chili garlic paste and stir again. Turn the stove off.

3. Beat the eggs in a separate container and pour into the steaming broth.

4. Stir together well and let sit for a moment to cook.

5. It's all done! Serve up some awesome tasting keto egg drop soup in only

5 minutes.

This makes 1 total serving of 5 Minute Keto Egg Drop Soup.

It comes out to be 279 Calories, 23g Fats, 2.5g Net Carbs, and 12g Protein.

CRISPY TOFU AND BOK CHOY SALAD

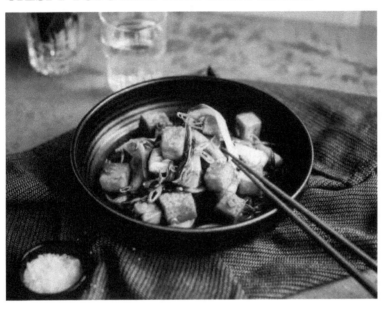

INGREDIENTS

Oven Baked Tofu

• 15 oz. Extra Firm Tofu

• 1 tbsp. Soy Sauce

• 1 tbsp. Sesame Oil

• 1 tbsp. Water

• 2 tsp. Minced Garlic

• 1 tbsp. Rice Wine Vinegar

- Juice 1/2 Lemon

Bok Choy Salad

- 9 oz. Bok Choy

- 1 stalk Green Onion

- 2 tbsp. Cilantro, chopped

- 3 tbsp. Coconut Oil

- 2 tbsp. Soy Sauce

- 1 tbsp. Sambal Olek

- 1 tbsp. Peanut Butter

- Juice 1/2 lime

- 7 drops Liquid Stevia

INSTRUCTION

1. Start by pressing the tofu. Lay the tofu in a kitchen towel and put something heavy over the top (like a cast iron skillet). It takes about 4-6 hours to dry out, and you may need to replace the kitchen towel half-way through.

2. Once the tofu is pressed, work on your marinade. Combine all of the in-

gredients for the marinade (soy sauce, sesame oil, water, garlic, vinegar, and lemon).

3. Chop the tofu into squares and place in a plastic bag along with the marinade. Let this marinate for at least 30 minutes, but preferably over night.

4. Pre-heat oven to 350F. Place tofu on a baking sheet lined with parchment

paper (or a silpat) and bake for 30-35 minutes.

5. As the tofu is cooked, get started on the bok choy salad. Chop cilantro and spring onion.

6. Mix all of the other ingredients together (except lime juice and bok choy) in a bowl. Then add cilantro and spring onion. Note: You can microwave coconut oil for 10-15 seconds to allow it it to melt.

7. Once the tofu is almost cooked, add lime juice into the salad dressing and

mix together.

8. Chop the bok choy into small slices, like you would cabbage.

9. Remove the tofu from the oven and assemble your salad with tofu, bok

choy, and sauce. Enjoy!

This makes a total of 3 servings of Crispy Tofu and Bok Choy Salad.

Each serving comes out to be 442 Calories, 35g Fats, 5.7g Net Carbs, and 25g Protein.

KETOGENIC NASI LEMAK

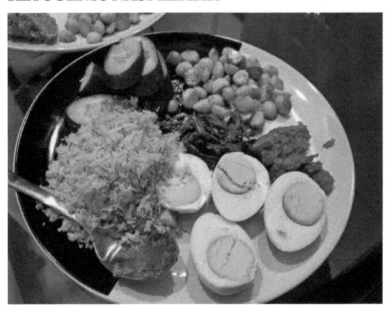

INGREDIENTS

Fried Chicken

• 2 boneless Chicken Thighs

• 1/2 tsp. Curry Powder

• 1/4 tsp. Turmeric Powder

• 1/2 tsp. Lime Juice

• 1/8 tsp. Salt

• 1/2 tsp. Coconut Oil

Nasi Lemak

- 3 tbsp. Coconut Milk (from the can)

- 3 slices Ginger

- 1/2 small Shallot, sliced

- 1/4 tsp. Salt (or to taste)

- 7 oz. riced Cauliflower

- 4 slices Cucumber

Fried Egg

- 1 large Egg

- 1/2 tbsp. Unsalted Butter

INSTRUCTION

1. Prepare 7 oz. cauliflower rice (by ricing cauliflower) and squeeze water out. Set aside.

2. Marinade 2 boneless Chicken Thighs with 1/2 tsp. Curry Powder, 1/4 tsp.

Turmeric Powder, 1/2 tsp. Lime Juice and 1/2 tsp. Salt. Set aside.

3. Prepare Sambal from this recipe on the website.

4. Fry the marinated chicken thighs until brown.

5. To prepare the rice, boil in a saucepan on medium heat: 3 tbsp. Coconut

Milk, 3 slices Ginger, 1/2 small Shallot and 1/4 tsp. Salt (or to taste). It should take about a minute or less.

6. Once bubbling, add in the riced Cauliflower and mix well.

7. Serve with 2 slices cucumber and a fried egg, along with 1 tbsp. Sambal and 1 piece Chicken Thigh.

This makes a total two servings of Nasi Lemak.

Each serving comes out to be 501.7 Calories, 39.9g Fats, 6.9g Net Carbs and 28.1g Protein.

LOW CARB SAUSAGE AND PEPPER SOUP

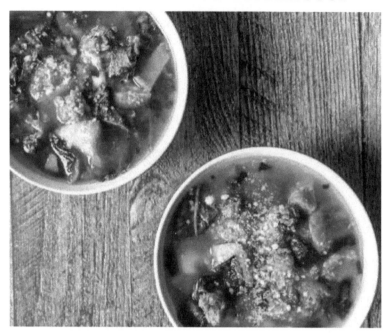

INGREDIENTS

- 32 oz. Pork Sausage

- 1 tbsp. Olive Oil

- 10 oz. Raw Spinach

- 1 medium Green Bell Pepper

- 1 can Tomatoes w/ Jalapenos

- 4 cups Beef Stock

- 1 tsp. Onion Powder

- 1 tbsp. Chili powder

- 1 tbsp. Cumin

- 1 tsp. Garlic Powder

- 1 tsp. Italian Seasoning

- 3/4 tsp. Kosher Salt

INSTRUCTION

1. Heat olive oil in a large pot over medium heat. Once hot, add sausage to the pan.

2. Once the sausage is seared on one side, mix it together to allow it to cook slightly.

3. As the sausage cooks, slice green pepper into pieces.

4. Add the peppers and stir everything together well. Season with salt and pepper.

5. Add the tomatoes and jalapenos from the can and stir once more.

6. Then, add the spinach on top of everything and place the lid on the pot.

7. Cook until spinach is wilted, about 6-7 minutes.

8. In the mean time, measure out all spices and grab your beef stock to have handy.

9. Once the spinach is wilted, mix it together with the sausage. Then add the spices and mix again. Lastly, add the broth and mix once again.

10. Replace the lid and cook for 30 minutes covered, reducing heat to medi-um-low.

11. Remove the lid from the pan and let simmer for 15 minutes longer.

This makes a total of 6 servings of Low Carb Sausage and Pepper Soup.

Each serving comes out to be 526 Calories, 43g Fats, 3.8g Net Carbs, and 27.8g Protein.

KETO PIGS IN A BLANKET

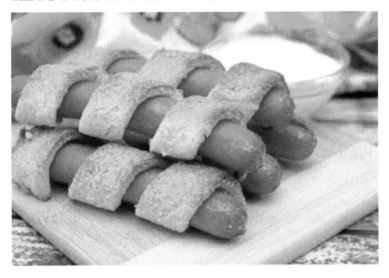

INGREDIENTS

• 37 Lit'l Smokies

• 8 oz. Cheddar Cheese (~2 cups)

• 3/4 cup Almond Flour

• 1 tbsp. Psyllium Husk Powder

• 1.5 oz. Cream Cheese (~3 tbsp.)

• 1 large Egg

• 1/2 tsp. Salt

• 1/2 tsp. Pepper

INSTRUCTION

1. Measure out the dry ingredients and the wet ingredients.

2. Start by melting the cheddar cheese in the microwave. Go in 20 second

intervals and stir to make sure the melting is even. once it's fully melted and slightly bubbling on the outside, it is ready.

3. While the cheddar is still hot, mix together all of the ingredients to make

the dough.

4. Spread the dough out on a silpat until it fills the entire sheet. Make sure it is even.

5. Place dough in the fridge to harden up for 15-20 minutes. Pre-heat your

oven to 400F while you do this.

6. Once the dough is cold, transfer to foil to cut. You should never use knives on your silpat.

7. Slice the dough into strips and wrap around the Lit'l Smokies. Then bake

for 13-15 minutes. Before taking them out, you can additionally broil them for 1-2 minutes.

8. Serve while warm. A sauce that is acidic and slightly sweet would work very well.

This makes 37 total Keto Pigs in a Blanket.

Each Pig in a Blanket comes out to be 72 Calories, 5.9g Fats, 0.6g Net Carbs, and 3.8g Protein.

BBQ BACON WRAPPED SMOKIES

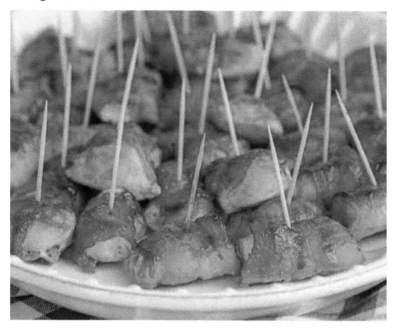

INGREDIENTS

• 24 Lit'l Smokies

• 6 slices Bacon

• 3 tbsp. Keto BBQ Sauce

• Salt and Pepper to taste

INSTRUCTION

1. Preheat oven to 375F. Start by chopping 6 slices of bacon into quarter-pie-ces. In total, you should have 24 quarter-slices of bacon. Place a little smokie on top of the slice of bacon.

2. Roll the little smokie up in the bacon so that there is a small amount of overlap.

3. Stick a toothpick into the overlapping piece and set on a cookie sheet cov-ered with foil.

4. Repeat the process for all of the smokies and place into the oven to bake for 25 minutes.

5. Take the smokies out of the oven and use a basting brush to brush BBQ sauce on the little smokies. They should be coated quite well.

6. Place back in the oven and bake for another 10-12 minutes.

7. Remove from the oven and let cool slightly.

8. Serve on a platter. Feel free to sprinkle some parmesan cheese and chopped spring onion over them.

This makes 4 servings of 6 BBQ Bacon Wrapped Smokies.

Each serving comes out to be 329 Calories, 28.5g Fats, 2.2g Net Carbs, and 13.5g Protein.

KETO ROTI JOHN

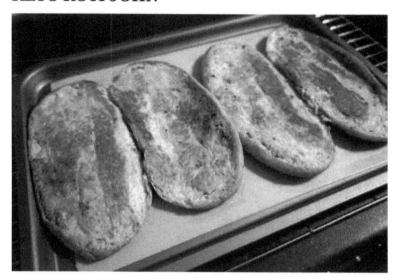

INGREDIENTS

The Bread

• 2 cups Mozzarella Cheese

• 3/4 cup Almond Flour

• 1 tbsp. Psyllium Husk Powder

• 3 tbsp. Cream Cheese

• 1 large Egg

• 1/2 tsp. Salt

• 1/2 tsp. Pepper

Omelette

• 1 tbsp. Coconut Oil

- 1/2 small Onion, diced

- 1 clove Garlic, finely chopped

- 1 tsp. Water

- 1/4 tsp. Curry Powder

- 4 tbsp. Ground Beef

- Salt and Pepper to Taste

- 2 1/2 tbsp. Unsalted Butter

- 2 large Eggs

- 2 tbsp. chopped Green Onion

- 2 tbsp. chopped Cilantro

- 2 tbsp. Mayonnaise (optional)

- 2 tbsp. Reduced Sugar Ketch up (or favorite sauce, optional)

- 5 slices Cucumber (garnish)

- 3 slices Tomatoes (garnish)

- 1 piece Butter Lettuce (garnish)

INSTRUCTION

1. Preheat oven to 400F. Follow the pizza base recipe for Low Carb Pepperoni Pizza, exclude the Italian Seasoning. Divide the dough into two. Shape each dough into a long bun, making sure both will fit on a large pan. Bake for about 30-40 minutes.

2. While waiting, preheat a pan on medium heat. Add in 1 tbsp. Coconut Oil. Once melted, saute the diced Onion. Once the onion turns translucent, add in the chopped Garlic. After 1 minute, add in 1/4 tsp. Curry Powder and 1 tsp. Water. Let the curry powder cook for 2 minutes.

3. Add in 4 tbsp. Ground Beef and cook until brown. Season with Salt and Pepper to taste. It should be cooked in such a way you would eat this on its own.

4. When the buns are ready, remove the buns from the oven. Cool both buns on a cooling rack. The buns should deflate a bit.

5. Once the buns become cool enough, slice them horizontally but not completely. Spread about 1/2 tbsp. of Unsalted Butter onto both buns.

6. Toast the buttered side of the buns with a pan.

7. In a mixing bowl, crack an egg. Add in about half of the cooked Ground Beef, 1 tbsp. each Green Onion and Cilantro. Season with a bit of Salt and Pepper. Mix well.

8. Preheat a large pan on medium heat. Melt 1 tbsp. of Unsalted Butter. Than, add in the omelette mixture to the pan.

9. Immediately cover the omelette with a bun.

10. When the omelette is cooked (after about 2-3 minutes), flip and toast the bun side until brown.

11. Remove from the pan and spread about 1 tbsp. of Mayonnaise and Reduced Sugar Ketchup (or any kinds of sauce) onto the omelette side. Garnish with some sliced Cucumber and Tomatoes, and Lettuce. Repeat steps 7-10 for the other bun.

12. Fold the buns and serve while hot!

This makes 4 total servings of Keto Roti John.

Each serving comes out to be 620 Calories, 53.3g Fats, 26g Protein, and 6.8g Net Carbs.

ROASTED RED BELL PEPPER AND CAULIFLOWER SOUP

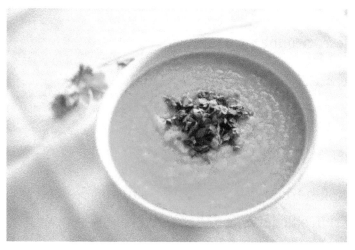

INGREDIENTS

• 2 medium Red Bell Peppers, cut in half and de-seeded

• 1/2 head Cauliflower, cut into florets

• 2 tbsp. Duck Fat

• 3 medium Green Onions, diced

• 3 cups Chicken Broth

• 1/2 cup Heavy Cream

• 4 tbsp. Duck Fat

• 1 tsp. Garlic Powder

- 1 tsp. Dried Thyme

- 1 tsp. Smoked Paprika

- 1/4 tsp. Red Pepper Flakes

- 4 oz. Goat Cheese, crumbled (to top)

- Salt and Pepper to Taste

INSTRUCTION

1. Put oven on broil setting. Slice peppers in half and de-seed them. Lay them skin side up on a foil-covered baking tray and broil for 10-15 minutes or until skin is charred and blackened.

2. While peppers are broiling, cut cauliflower into florets. If the florets are large, cut florets in half or quarters.

3. Once peppers are done, remove from oven and place in a container with a lid, or a food saver bag and seal. Let the peppers steam and cook longer to soften while cauliflower roasts.

4. Use 2 tbsp. melted duck fat, salt, and pepper to season the cauliflower. Roast cauliflower in 400F oven for 30-35 minutes.

5. Remove the skins from the peppers by peeling it off carefully.

6. In a pot, bring 4 tbsp. duck fat to heat and add diced green onion. Once green onion is slightly cooked, add seasonings into the pan to toast.

7. Add chicken broth, red pepper, and cauliflower to the pan. Let this simmer for 10-20 minutes.

8. Take an immersion blender to the mixture. Make sure that all fats are emul-sified with the mixture by the time you're finished – about 1-2 minutes. Season to taste, then add cream and mix.

9. Serve with some crispy bacon and goats cheese. Garnish with extra thyme and green onion.

This makes 5 total servings of Roasted Red Bell Pepper & Cauliflower Soup.

Each serving comes out to be 345 Calories, 32g Fats, 6.2g Net Carbs, and 6.4g Protein.

SOUTHWESTERN PORK STEW

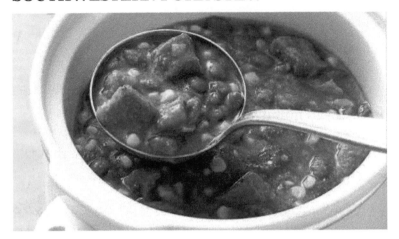

INGREDIENTS

• 1 lb. Cooked Pork Shoulder, sliced

• 2 tsp. Chili Powder

• 2 tsp. Cumin

• 1 tsp. Minced Garlic

• 1/2 tsp. Salt

• 1/2 tsp. Pepper

• 1 tsp. Paprika

• 1 tsp. Oregano

• 1/4 tsp. Cinnamon

• 2 Bay Leafs

• 6 oz. Button Mushrooms

- 1/2 sliced Jalapeno

- 1/2 medium Onion

- 1/2 Green Bell Pepper, sliced

- 1/2 Red Bell Pepper, sliced

- Juice 1/2 Lime (to finish)

- 2 cups Gelatinous Bone Broth

- 2 cup Chicken Broth

- 1/2 cup Strong Coffee

- 1/4 cup Tomato Paste

INSTRUCTION

1. Prep all vegetables by slicing and chopping them.

2. Let your bone broth start to come to room temperature.

3. Bring a pan to high heat with 2 tbsp. Olive Oil. Once hot, add vegetables

and saute them until they are slightly cooked and aromatic.

4. Measure out all spices into a small container so you can use them as needed.

5. Slice pork (preferably a tougher meat for this) into bite size chunks.

6. Add bone broth, chicken broth, and coffee to slow cooker.

7. Add pork and mushrooms to the slow cooker and mix together.

8. Add spices and vegetables (with oil) to the slow cooker. Mix together well, cover, and set on low for 4-10 hours.

9. Once it's finished, take the lid off and stir together.

10. Serve it up!

This makes a total of 4 servings.

Each serving comes out to be 386 Calories, 28.9g Fats, 6.4g Net Carbs, and 19.9g Protein.

Feel free to add butter or sour cream on the finish to extra fats.

CHICKEN ENCHILADA SOUP

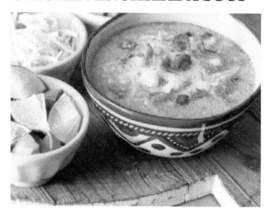

INGREDIENTS

- 3 tbsp. Olive Oil

- 3 stalks Celery, diced

- 1 medium Red Bell Pepper, diced

- 2 tsp. Garlic, minced

- 4 cups Chicken Broth

- 1 cup Diced Tomatoes

- 8 oz. Cream Cheese

- 6 oz. Chicken, shredded

- 2 tsp. Cumin

- 1 tsp. Oregano

- 1 tsp. Chili Powder

- 1/2 tsp. Cayenne Pepper

- 1/2 cup Cilantro, chopped

- 1/2 medium Lime, juiced

- Salt and Pepper to Taste

INSTRUCTION

1. Dice 3 stalks of celery (cut the tips off of each end) and 1 medium red bell

pepper. Mince the 2 tsp. of garlic (about 2 cloves) and get your cilantro out.

2. In a pot, heat 3 tbsp. olive oil over medium high heat.

3. Once the oil is hot, add celery, pepper, and garlic. Let this cook until the

celery softens. Add salt and pepper to taste.

4. Once celery is cooked, add 1 cup Diced Tomatoes and stir well. Let this

cook for about 2-3 minutes.

5. Add spices and additional salt and pepper if needed. Stir this up and leave for a 1-2 minutes.

6. In the mean time, chop up the cilantro (make sure you cut the stems off).

7. You'll need about 1/2 cup in total.

8. Add 4 cups chicken broth and cilantro to the pan. Stir everything together.

9. Bring the soup up to a boil and then reduce heat to low. Let this simmer for 20 minutes.

10. Measure out the cream cheese and add it to the pan. Stir in well and bring to a boil again. Once boiling, turn to low and simmer for 20-25 minutes.

11. Shred the chicken with a fork. You can either cook this fresh as you're making the soup or you can use leftover rotisserie chicken.

12. Once simmered, add chicken to the pan and squeeze the lime juice over the top. Stir together until everything is mixed.

13. Serve up with extra limes and sour cream! You can additionally garnish with shredded cheese, extra bell pepper, or fresh cilantro.

This makes 4 total servings.

Each serving comes out to 345 Calories, 31.3g Fats, 6g Net Carbs, and 13.3g Protein.

THAI PEANUT SHRIMP CURRY

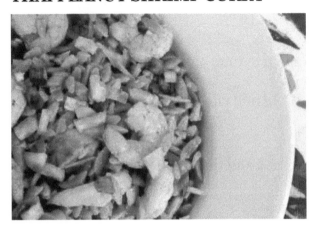

INGREDIENTS

- 2 tbsp. Green Curry Paste

- 1 cup Vegetable Stock

- 1 cup Coconut Milk

- 6 oz. Pre-cooked Shrimp

- 5 oz. Broccoli Florets

- 3 tbsp. Cilantro, chopped

- 2 tbsp. Coconut Oil

- 1 tbsp. Peanut Butter

- 1 tbsp. Soy Sauce (or coconut aminos)

- Juice of 1/2 Lime

- 1 medium Spring Onion, chopped

- 1 tsp. Crushed Roasted Garlic

- 1 tsp. Minced Ginger

- 1 tsp. Fish Sauce

- 1/2 tsp. Turmeric

- 1/4 tsp. Xanthan Gum

- 1/2 cup Sour Cream (for topping)

INSTRUCTION

1. Start by adding 2 tbsp. coconut oil in a pan over medium heat.

2. When the coconut oil is melted and the pan is hot, add the 1 tsp. roasted

garlic, 1 tsp. minced ginger, and 1 spring onion (chopped). Allow to cook for

about a minute, then add 1 tbsp. green curry paste, and 1/2 tsp. turmeric.

3. Add 1 tbsp. soy sauce (or coconut aminos), 1 tsp. fish sauce, and 1 tbsp.

peanut butter to the pan and mix together well.

4. Add 1 cup of vegetable stock and 1 cup of coconut milk (from the carton).

Stir well and then add another 1 tbsp. green curry paste.

5. Let simmer for a few minutes. In the mean time, measure out 6 oz. pre-

cooked shrimp.

6. Add 1/4 tsp. xanthan gum to the curry and mix well.

7. Once your curry begins thickening up a little bit, add the broccoli florets

and stir well.

8. Chop 3 tbsp. fresh cilantro and add to the pan.

9. Finally, once you are happy with the consistency of the curry, add the shrimp and lime juice from 1/2 lime, and mix everything together.

10. Let simmer for a few minutes. Taste and season with salt and pepper if needed.

11. Serve! You can stir in 1/4 cup of sour cream per serving.

This makes 2 servings of Thai Peanut Shrimp Curry.

Each serving comes out to be 455 Calories, 31.5g Fats, 8.9g Net Carbs, and 27g Protein.

KETO GRILLED CHEESE SANDWICH

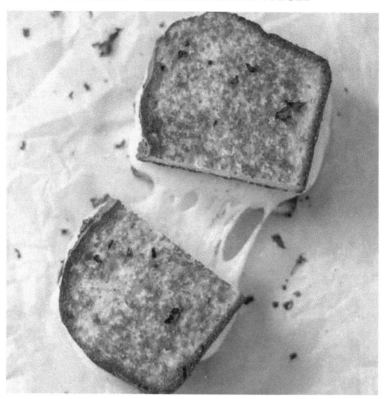

INGREDIENTS

Bun Ingredients

• 2 large Eggs

• 2 tbsp. Almond Flour

• 1 1/2 tbsp. Psyllium Husk Powder

- 1/2 tsp. Baking Powder

- 2 tbsp. Soft Butter

Fillings & Extras

- 2 oz. Cheddar Cheese (or white cheddar, if you're feeling frisky)

- 1 tbsp. Butter, for frying

INSTRUCTION

1. Let 2 tbsp. butter come to room temperature in a mug. Once it's soft, add

2 tbsp. Almond Flour, 1 1/2 tbsp. Psyllium Husk, and 1/2 tsp. Baking Powder.

2. Mix this together as well as you can so that a thick dough is formed.

3. Add 2 large eggs and continue mixing together. You want a dough that is pretty thick. If your dough isn't thick, continue mixing the dough – it will thicken up as you mix it (this can take up to 60 seconds).

4. Pour the dough into a square container or bowl. Level it off and clean off the sides that that it comes out as level as you can get it.

5. Microwave for about 90-100 seconds. You will have to check the do-ne-ness of it to make sure it doesn't need longer.

6. Remove from the container or bowl by flipping it upside down and lightly tapping the bottom. Cut it in half using a bread knife.

7. Measure out the cheese you can and stick it between the buns.

8. Bring 1 tbsp. butter to heat in a pan over medium heat. Once hot, add bun and allow to cook in the butter. This should be absorbed by the bread as you cook and give a delicious, crisp outside.

9. Serve up with a side salad for some delicious ooey-gooey grilled cheese!

This will make 1 Keto Grilled Cheese Sandwich.

For the sandwich, it comes out to 793 Calories, 70g Fats, 4.7g Net Carbs, and 29g Protein.

FRESH BELL PEPPER BASIL PIZZA

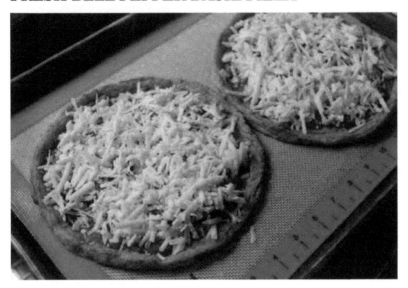

INGREDIENTS

Pizza Base

• 6 oz. Mozzarella Cheese

• 1/2 cup Almond Flour

• 2 tbsp. Psyllium Husk

• 2 tbsp. Cream Cheese

• 2 tbsp. Fresh Parmesan

Cheese

• 1 large Egg

- 1 tsp. Italian Seasoning

- 1/2 tsp. Salt

- 1/2 tsp. Pepper

Toppings

- 4 oz. Shredded Cheddar
Cheese

- 1 medium Vine Tomato

- 1/4 cup Rao's Tomato Sauce

- 2/3 medium Bell Pepper

- 2-3 tbsp. Fresh Chopped Basil

INSTRUCTION

1. Preheat oven to 400F. Start by measuring out all of your dry spices and flours in a bowl. 1/2 cup Almond Flour, 2 tbsp. Psyllium Husk, 2 tbsp. Fresh Parmesan Cheese, 1 tsp. Italian Seasoning, 1/2 tsp. Salt, and 1/2 tsp. Pepper.

2. Measure out 6 oz. Mozzarella Cheese into a bowl.

3. Microwave the cheese for 40-50 seconds until it's completely melted and pliable with your hands. Add 2 tbsp. Cream Cheese to the top.

4. Add 1 egg to the dry ingredients and mix together a little bit.

5. Add the melted mozzarella cheese and cream cheese to the egg and dry ingredients and mix everything together. Don't mind getting your hands dirty here – they'll be the best tool for the job. You'll get a bit messy, but it'll be oh so worth it in the end.

6. Break the dough into 2 equal (or almost equal) portions. Roll the doughout quite thin – a little under 1/4. Here, you can use the top of a pot or other large round object to cut out your pizza base. You can form the circles by hand, but

7. Fold the edges of the dough inward and form a small crust on the dough. If you have any scraps remaining, you can add it into the crust if you want.

8. Bake the dough for 10 minutes. Just enough so they're starting to get slightly golden brown.

9. Remove the crust from the oven and let cool for a moment.

10. Slice a medium vine tomato and put half on each pizza along with 2 tbsp.

11. Rao's tomato sauce per pizza. Aww...they look like little peace signs.

12. Top these suckers with cheese – about 2 oz. Shredded Cheddar per pizza.

13. Chop up the bell peppers. You can use 1 bell pepper or 2 different colors.

14. Arrange the peppers how you like and throw it back in the oven for another 8-10 minutes.

15. Remove the pizzas from the oven and let cool. In the meantime, slice up some fresh basil and have it ready for serving.

16. Serve it up – top with fresh basil and enjoy the fresh bites of summer!

This makes 2 pizzas.

Per 1/2 of a pizza, this is 410 Calories, 31.3g Fats, 5.3g Net Carbs, and 24.8g Protein.

LOW CARB PASTA A LA CARBONARA

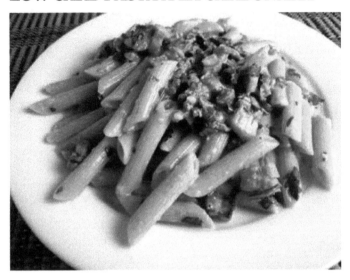

INGREDIENTS

• 2/3 Pasta Recipe from Keto-fied!

• 5 Oz. Bacon

• 2 large Egg Yolks

• 1 large Egg

• 1 tbsp. Heavy Cream

• 1/3 cup Fresh Grated

Parmesan (Plus garnish)

• 3 tbsp. Fresh Chopped Basil

• Fresh Ground Black Pepper to Taste

INSTRUCTION

1. Prepare pasta as described in Keto-fied: Comfort Food Made Low Carb.

2. Freeze bacon for 15 minutes prior for easier cutting. Slice bacon into small cubes and cook until crisp over high heat.

3. Set bacon aside to cool on paper towels and become even crispier.

4. Save 1/3 bacon grease and keep other 2/3 in the pan. Mix together 1 large egg and 2 large egg yolks.

5. Measure out 1/3 cup freshly grated parmesan cheese.

6. Add parmesan, cream, and saved 1/3 bacon grease that was saved to the egg and egg yolk mixture. Stir together well until a thick sauce is formed.

7. Cook pasta in a pan with the bacon grease that is left over high heat.

8. Add pasta to a mixing bowl, then add crisped bacon and toss.

9. Add carbonara sauce to the pasta along with 2 tbsp. freshly chopped basil and fresh cracked black pepper. Mix together until all strands of pasta is covered completely.

10. Garnish with extra fresh cracked black pepper and chopped basil.

This makes 3 total servings of Low Carb Pasta a la Carbonara.

Per serving, it comes out to 553 Calories, 44g Fats, 3.8g Net Carbs, and 21.7g Protein.

A perfectly ketogenic meal that includes delicious and realistic tasting pasta!

SPICY JALAPENO POPPERS

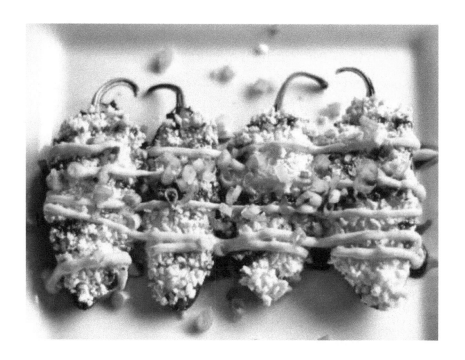

INGREDIENTS

- 5 OZ. Cream Cheese

- 1/4 cup Mozzarella Cheese

- 8 medium Jalapeno Peppers

- 1/4 tsp. Salt

- 1/4 tsp. Pepper

- 1/2 tsp. Mrs. Dash Table Blend

- 8 slices Bacon

INSTRUCTION

1. Preheat oven to 400F. Wash all of your jalapeno peppers. Foil a baking sheet and remove the stems of your peppers

2. Slice each pepper in half, making sure that it is an even cut on each pepper.

3. Using a spoon, scrape out all of the guts of the peppers. You can leave a few seeds inside for extra heat if you'd like.

4. In a bowl, combine 5 oz. Cream Cheese, 1/4 cup Mozzarella Cheese, and spices of your choice. Also use 1/4 tsp. Salt, 1/4 tsp. Pepper, and 1/2 tsp. A Dash Table Blend.

5. Pack the cream cheese mixture into each pepper, creating a mound that the other half will fit on top of.

6. Press the other half of the peppers into the cream cheese mixture, closing the peppers up like they were never cut.

7. Wrap each pepper in bacon, starting from the bottom and working your way up to the top.

8. Bake for 20-25 minutes or until bacon begins it crisp up and is cooked completely. Broil for additional 2-3 minutes to get a darker color and more crisp on the bacon.

9. Serve up – serve with a saute of broccoli, red pepper, and celery in the leftover bacon fat from the baking sheet.

This makes 8 Spicy Jalapeno Poppers.

Each jalapeno popper comes out to 182 Calories, 16.5g Fats, 1.3g Net Carbs, and 4.8g Protein.

ASIAN CUCUMBER SALAD

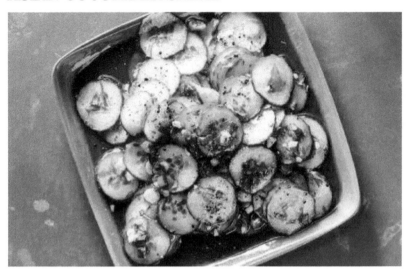

INGREDIENTS

- 3/4 large Cucumber

- 1 packet Shiritaki Noodles

- 2 tbsp. Coconut Oil

- 1 medium Spring Onion

- 1/4 tsp. Red Pepper Flakes

- 1 tbsp. Sesame Oil

- 1 tbsp. Rice Vinegar

- 1 tsp. Sesame Seeds

- Salt and Pepper to Taste

INSTRUCTION

1. Remove shiritaki noodles from the package and rise off completely. This may take a few minutes, but make sure that all of the extra water that came in its package is washed off.

2. Set noodles on a kitchen towel and thoroughly dry them.

3. Bring 2 tbsp. Coconut Oil to medium-high heat in a pan.

4. Once the oil is hot, add noodles and cover (it will splatter). Let these fry for 5-7 minutes or until crisp and browned.

5. Remove shiritaki noodles from the pan and set on paper towels to cool and dry.

6. Slice cucumber thin and arrange on a plate in the design you'd like.

7. Add 1 medium Spring Onion, 1/4 tsp. Red Pepper Flakes, 1 tbsp. Sesame Oil, 1 tbsp. Rice Vinegar, 1 tsp. Sesame Seeds, and Salt and Pepper to taste. You can also pour over the coconut oil from the pan you fried the noodles in. This will add a salty component so keep that in mind. Store this in the fridge for at least 30 minutes before serving!

This yields 1 serving, which comes out to 416 Caloies, 43g Fats, 7g Net Carbs, and 2g Protein.

LOW CARB MOROCCAN MEATBALLS

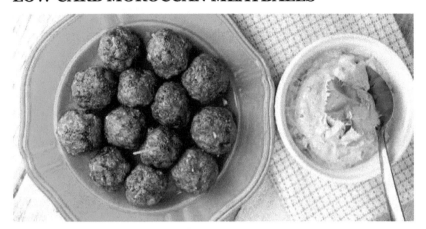

INGREDIENTS

Low Carb Moroccan Meatballs

• 1 lb. Ground Lamb

• 1 tbsp. Finely Chopped Fresh Mint

• 1 tbsp. Finely Chopped Fresh Cilantro

• 2 tsp. Fresh Thyme

• 1 tsp. Minced Garlic

• 1 tsp. Ground Coriander

• 1 tsp. Kosher Salt

• 1 tsp. Ground Cumin

• 1/2 tsp. Onion Powder

• 1/2 tsp. Allspice

- 1/4 tsp. Paprika

- 1/4 tsp. Oregano

- 1/4 tsp. Curry Powder

- 1/4 tsp. Freshly Ground Black Pepper

Faux Yogurt Sauce

- 1/2 cup Coconut Cream

- 2 tbsp. Coconut Water

- 1 1/4 tsp. Cumin

- 1 tbsp. Finely Chopped Fresh Cilantro

- 1 tbsp. Finely Chopped Fresh Mint

- Zest 1/2 Lemon

- 1 tsp. Lemon Juice

- 1/4 tsp. Salt

INSTRUCTION

1. Preheat oven to 350F. Finely chop 1 tbsp. fresh mint, 1 tbsp. fresh cilantro, and 2 tsp. Fresh Thyme.

2. Break up the ground lamb, then add the chopped spices plus 1 tsp. Minced Garlic, 1 tsp. Ground Coriander, 1 tsp. Kosher Salt, 1 tsp. Ground Cumin, 1/2 tsp. Onion Powder, 1/2 tsp. Allspice, 1/4

tsp. Paprika, 1/4 tsp. Oregano, 1/4 tsp. Curry Powder and 1/4 tsp. Freshly Ground Black Pepper.

3. Mix together the mixture well so that all of the spices are evenly distributed.

4. Roll the meat into 15-18 meatballs. You can alternatively make larger meat-balls if you want to make this an entree. Put the meatballs in the oven for 15-18 minutes or until the center is no longer pink.

5. While meatballs are baking, measure out 1/2 cup coconut cream from the top of a can of coconut milk.

6. Add 2 tbsp. coconut water from underneath the cream in the can. Then, add 1 1/4 tsp. Cumin, 1 tbsp. Finely Chopped Cilantro, 1 tbsp. Finely Chopped Mint.

7. Mix the sauce well, then zest 1/2 lemon and add 1 tsp. lemon juice. Mix well.

8. Let the meatballs cool for a moment before serving. Optional: Add runoff fats from the meatballs into the sauce and mix well.

9. Serve with faux yogurt sauce on the side!

This made a total of 18 meatballs, which came out to about 4 servings. Each serving comes out to be 399 Calories, 32.5g Fats, 3g Net Carbs, and 19.5g Protein.

PORTOBELLO PERSONAL PIZZAS

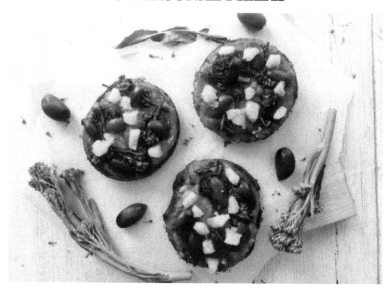

INGREDIENTS

- 4 large Portobello Mushroom Caps

- 1 medium Vine Tomato

- 4 oz. Fresh Mozzarella Cheese

- 1/4 cup Fresh Chopped Basil

- 6 tbsp. Olive Oil

- 20 slices Pepperoni

- Salt and Pepper to Taste

INSTRUCTION

1. Get your 4 portobello mushrooms ready.

2. Scrape out all of the innards of the mushroom. Then dig into the flesh and get the mushroom about 1cm thick.

3. Set the oven to broil on high and rub the insides of each mushroom with

just under 1 tbsp. Olive Oil. You should use 3 tbsp. Olive Oil between the 4

mushrooms. Season with salt and pepper to taste.

4. Broil the mushroom for about 4-5 minutes.

5. Flip the mushrooms over and rub again with 3 tbsp. Olive Oil. Season with salt and pepper to taste. Broil the mushrooms with the other side facing up for about 3-4 minutes longer.

6. Slice a tomato thin, about 12-16 slices in total. Chop 1/4 cup basil into strips.

7. Lay the tomato and basil into each mushroom. depending on how many slices of tomato, you will put 3-4 slices in each mushroom. About 1 tbsp. of

basil on top of each mushroom also.

8. Lay 5 slices of pepperoni onto each mushroom and top with fresh cubed mozzarella cheese (1 oz per mushroom).

9. Broil again for 2-4 minutes, or until cheese is melted and starts to brown.

10. Serve up!

This makes 4 total Portobello Pizzas.

Per Pizza it is 321 Calories, 31g Fats, 2.8g Net Carbs, and 8.5g Protein.

KETO THAI CHICKEN FLATBREAD PIZZA

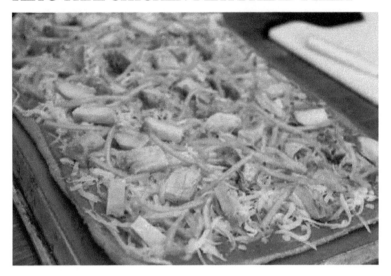

DINNER

INGREDIENTS

Peanut Sauce

• 4 tbsp. PBFit

• 2 tbsp. Rice Wine Vinegar

• 4 tbsp. Soy Sauce

• 4 tbsp. Reduced Sugar Ketchup

• 4 tbsp. Coconut Oil

• 1 tsp. Fish Sauce

• Juice of 1/2 Lime

Pizza Base

- 2 cups Mozzarella Cheese (~8 oz.)

- 3/4 cup Almond Flour

- 1 tbsp. Psyllium Husk Powder

- 3 tbsp. Cream Cheese (~1.5 oz.)

- 1 large Egg

- 1/2 tsp. Onion Powder

- 1/2 tsp. Garlic Powder

- 1/2 tsp. Ginger Powder

- 1/2 tsp. Salt

- 1/2 tsp. Pepper

Toppings

- 2 small Chicken Thighs, cooked

- 3 oz. Mung Bean Sprouts

- 6 oz. Mozzarella Cheese

- 2 medium Green Onions

- 1 1/2 oz. Shredded Carrot

- 2 tbsp. Peanuts, chopped

- 3 tbsp. Cilantro, chopped

INSTRUCTION

1. Pre-heat oven to 400F. First combine all of the ingredients for the sauce. Use an immersion blender if you need to to emulsify the coconut oil into the sauce. I didn't have too big an issue because I was using melted coconut oil.

2. Get the ingredients ready for the base of your pizza. The mozzarella and cream cheese in one bowl, then all of the dry ingredients in another. Micro-wave the cheese for about 1 minute on high or until it's melted and bubbling on the sides.

3. Add the egg to the cheese and mix together well. Then, add the dry ingre-dients into the cheese and thoroughly mix.

4. On a silpat, press the pizza base from edge to edge, creating a large rect-angle the size of a cookie sheet.

5. Put the pizza in the oven for about 12-14 minutes, or until it's nice and browned on the top.

6. Chop the pre-cooked chicken into bite sized chunks and set aside.

7. Flip the pizza over so that the bottom is now facing the top.

8. Top the pizza with the sauce, chicken, shredded carrots, and mozzarella. Place back into the oven for 7-10 minutes, or until cheese is nice and melted.

9. Top with mung bean sprouts, chopped spring onion, chopped peanuts and cilantro to taste.

This makes 12 total slices of Keto Thai Chicken Pizza.

Each slice comes out to be 268 Calories, 21g Fats, 3.2g Net Carbs, and 15g Protein.

REVERSE SEARED RIBEYE STEAK

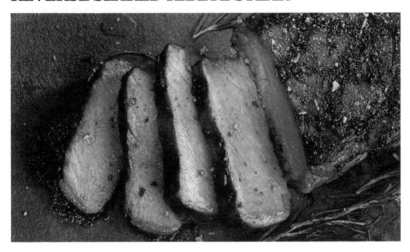

DINNER

INGREDIENTS

• 2 medium Ribeye Steaks (~1.2 lbs.)

• 3 tbsp. Bacon Fat (or other high smoke point oil)

• Salt and Pepper to Taste

INSTRUCTION

1. Preheat oven to 250F. Put your steaks on a wire rack on top of a cookie sheet. Season heavily with salt and pepper on all sides of the meat.

2. Stick an instant-read thermometer through the side of the steak so that the tip reaches the middle. Set thermometer for

123F internal temperature and bake in the oven until internal temperature is reached. About 40-45 minutes.

3. Let the steaks rest for a few minutes. Usually only a few minutes. The juices won't run as much with this method because it's cooking low and slow, rather than a fast sear.

4. Heat the bacon grease in a cast iron skillet or cermic cast iron skillet and wait until the pan is very hot. I normally wait until the smoke point of the grease is hit. Place the steaks in and sear for 30 – 45 seconds on each side.

5. Don't forget to sear the sides of the steak!

6. Let rest for 2-3 minutes and serve warm. Enjoy! Feel free to serve up with some awesome and super Easy Creamy Cauliflower Mashed Potatoes.

This makes a total of 3 servings of Reverse Seared Ribeye Steak.

Each ~6.5 oz. serving comes out to be 430 Calories, 31.7g Fats, 0g Net Carbs, and 30.3g Protein.

KETO TATER TOT NACHOS (AKA TOTCHOS)

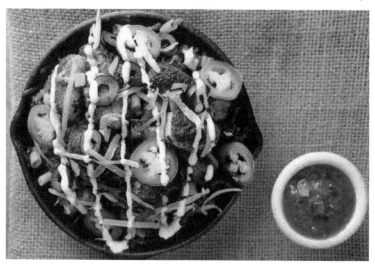

DINNER

INGREDIENTS

- 2 servings Keto Tater Tots

- 6 oz. Ground Beef (80/20), cooked

- 2 oz. Cheddar Cheese, shredded

- 2 tbsp. Sour Cream

- 6 Black Olives, sliced

- 1 tbsp. Salsa

- 1/2 medium Jalapeno Pepper, sliced

INSTRUCTION

1. In a small casserole dish or mini cast iron skillet, lay down 9-10 keto tater tots .

2. Add 1/2 ground beef, and 1/2 of the shredded cheese. Start the second layer with less tater tots, 1/2 of the remaining beef, and 1/2 of the remaining cheese. Repeat with the last of the tater tots. Broil in the oven for 4-5 minutes so that the cheese melts.

3. Serve with jalapenos, sour cream, black olives, and salsa. Enjoy

This makes 2 total servings of Keto Tater Tot Nachos (AKA Totchos).

Each serving comes out to be637 Calories, 52.5g Fats, 5.5g Net Carbs, and 32.3g Protein

BLACKBERRY CHIPOTLE CHICKEN WING

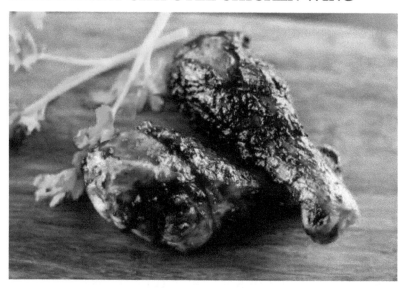

DINNER

INGREDIENTS

• 3 lbs. Chicken Wings (~20 wings, butchered)

• 1/2 cup Blackberry Chipotle Jam

• 1/2 cup Water

• Salt and Pepper to Taste

INSTRUCTION

1. Start by butchering the chicken wings. Place the chicken wing down on a cutting board and let the "V" naturally occur. Cut into the V, allowing your kni-fe to do most of the work. You should only be cutting through cartilage, and not bone.

2. Once you have the drummette detached from the wing, locate the sec-ondary "V" that occurs between the wing and the wing tip. Use the weight of your knife to cut the wing tip off. You can freeze these to make bone broth with later.

3. In a bowl, combine 1/2 cup Blackberry Chipotle Jam and 1/2 cup water. Whisk to combine, then add 2/3 marinade with the chicken wings and salt and pepper in a plastic bag. Let this sit for at least 30 minutes, or up to overnight.

4. In the meantime, preheat oven to 400F. Once the chicken is finished mar-inating, lay on a cookie sheet with a wire rack on top. Bake for 15 minutes at 400F, then flip and turn oven up to 425F. Brush the remaining marinade over each wing (now the bottom side) and bake for an additional 20-30 minutes, or until wings are cris

5. Remove from the oven, let cool, and enjoy!

This makes a total of 20 Blackberry Chipotle Chicken Wings.

Per 4 wings, it comes out to be 503 Calories, 39.1g Fats, 1.8g Net Carbs, and 34.5g Protein.

KETO CHICKEN PAD THAI

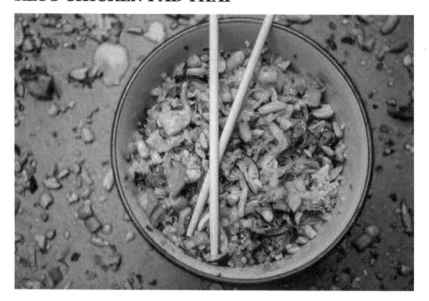

D I N N E R

INGREDIENTS

Pad Thai Sauce

• Juice 1/2 Lime

• Juice 1/3 Lemon

1/2 tbsp. Reduced Sugar

Ketchup

• 1/2 tsp. Worcestershire

Sauce

- 3 tbsp. Red Boat Fish Sauce

1 1/2 tbsp. Sambal Olek

1 1/2 tsp. Minced Garlic

- 1 tbsp. Natural Peanut Butter

- 1 tsp. Rice Wine Vinegar

- 7 drops Liquid Stevia

Noodles and Toppings

- 1/4 cup Cilantro, chopped

- 3 medium Green Onions, chopped

- 2 large Eggs

- 2 packets Shirataki Noodles (House Foods Tofu Shirataki)

- 3 medium Chicken Thighs lbs. deskinned and deboned

- 4 tbsp. Coconut Oil

- 4 oz. Mung Bean Sprouts

- 2 tbsp. Peanuts, chopped

INSTRUCTION

1. Mix together all of the ingredients for the sauce using a fork or whisk. Set aside.

2. Drain shirataki noodles and rinse well with hot water. Do this about 5 or 6 times, then dry as much as you can using a cloth.

3. To get out extra moisture from the noodles, wring them out using a kitchen towel. Wring them out as much as possible to get rid of the excess moisture.

4. Debone chicken thighs. Start by cutting a line in the chicken where the bone is using kitchen shears. Cut all of the meat away from the bone, then remove by the bone by cutting around each end.

5. Once the chicken thighs are deboned, remove the skin (this can be done with your hand), and cut into cubed pieces.

6. Heat 2 tbsp. Coconut Oil in a pan over medium-high heat. Once the pan is hot, add the chicken to create a sear. Make sure not to overcrowd the pan.

7. Flip the chicken pieces over to create a sear on the other side. Remove chicken from the pan (including the oil), and repeat using more coconut oil. Set chicken aside in a bowl.

8. Chop green onion and cilantro so that you're ready to use it.

9. In the same pan you used to cook the chicken, add the shirataki noodles and dry fry them for 5-8 minutes or until noodles become firmer to the touch.

10. Reduce heat of the pan, and add 2 eggs that have been whisked into the noodles. Mix together so that the eggs become scrambled and broken apart.

11. Finally, add the sauce, chicken (including all of the oil), cilantro, and green onion to the noodles. Let this cook down for about 5-10 minutes depending on thickness you want.

12. Serve with mung bean sprouts, and chopped peanuts over the top. Garnish with extra cilantro, green onion, and red pepper flakes.

This makes a total of 4 servings of Keto Chicken Pad Thai.

Each serving comes out to be 431 Calories, 35.3g Fats, 5g Net Carbs, and 26.3g Protein.

LOW-CARB CHICKEN CURRY

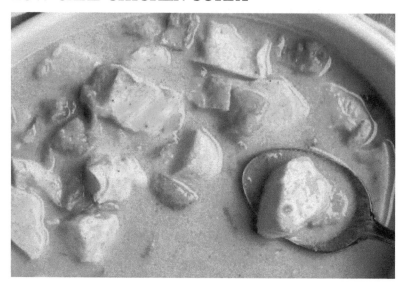

DINNER

INGREDIENTS

- 2 tbsp. Coconut Oil

- 1.5 inch Ginger

- 1 medium Green Chilli

- 2 small Shallots

- 2 cloves Garlic

- 2 tsp. Turmeric Powder

- 1 stalk Lemongrass

- 1/2 cup Coconut Milk (from the can)

- 1/2 cup Water

- 6 small Chicken Drumsticks (~21 oz. bone-in)

- 1/2 tsp. Salt

- 1 tbsp. Cilantro, chopped

INSTRUCTION

1. Bruise 1 stalk Lemongrass. This will help release the aroma when cooking.

2. With a pestle and mortar, pound 1.5 inch Ginger, 1 Green Chilli, 2 Shallots and 2 cloves Garlic. Alternatively, you can use a blender.

3. In a pre-heated pot over medium heat, melt 2 tbsp. Coconut Oil. Once hot, add in the pounded ingredients and saute.

4. After 3-4 minutes, add in 2 tsp. Turmeric Powder and the smashed Lemon grass and saute once again.

5. Add in Chicken meat and mix well with the sauteed ingredients.

6. Once the meat is coated, pour in 1/2 cup each Coconut Milk and Water.

7. Add in 1/2 tsp. Salt and cover the pot. Let everything cook for about 20 minutes or until desired thickness is reached and chicken is cooked through.

8. Sprinkle 1 tbsp. chopped Cilantro over the top and serve!

This makes a total of 3 servings of Low-Carb Chicken Curry.

Each serving comes out to be 493 Calories, 35g Protein, 4.8g Net Carbs, and 37.5g Protein.

THAI CHICKEN ZOODLES

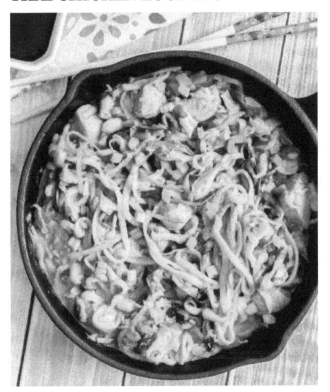

D I N N E R

INGREDIENTS

- 1/2 tsp. Curry Powder

- 3.5 oz. Chicken Thigh

- 1 tbsp. Unsalted Butter

- 1 tbsp. Coconut Oil

- 1 stalk Spring Onion

- 1 clove Garlic

- 1 large Egg

- 1.4 oz. Bean Sprouts

- 3.5 oz. Zucchini

- 1 tsp. Soy Sauce (or Coconut Aminos)

- 1/2 tsp. Oyster Sauce

- 1/8 tsp. White Pepper

- 1 tsp. Lime Juice

- Red Chilies, chopped

- Salt and Pepper to Taste

INSTRUCTION

1. Season the Chicken with 1/2 tsp. Curry Powder and a pinch of Salt and Pe-pper. Keep aside for a while.

2. Prepare the sauce by combining 1 tsp. Soy Sauce, 1/2 tsp. Oyster Sauce, and 1/8 tsp. White Pepper.

3. Finely chop Spring Onion and Garlic and make Zoodles out of Zucchini. You can use the spiralizer to do so.

4. Fry the seasoned Chicken with 1 tbsp. Unsalted Butter until brown. When done, slice to bite-sized pieces.

5. In the same pan, melt 1 tbsp. Coconut Oil on high heat. Saute chopped Spring Onion until fragrant.

6. Add chopped Garlic and again saute until fragrant.

7. Crack an Egg into the pan and make a scrambled egg. Saute until slightly brown.

8. Add in Bean Sprouts and Zoodles. Mix everything well together.

9. Add in the sauce and stir. Reduce until there is little liquid left.

10. Add in the fried Chicken pieces and stir.

11. Garnish with a few chopped Red Chilies and squeeze some Lime Juice on top. Serve while hot!

This makes 1 serving of Thai Chicken Zoodles.

The serving comes out to be 580 Calories, 49.1g Fats, 6.8g Net Carbs, and 25.8g Protein.

ULTIMATE KETO COFFEE CAKE

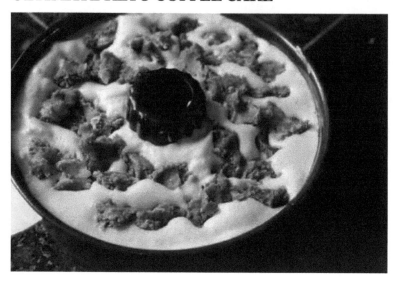

INGREDIENTS

Base

• 6 Large Eggs, Separated

• 6 Oz. Cream Cheese

• 1/4 Cup Erythritol

• 1/4 tsp. Liquid Stevia

• 1/4 Cup Unflavored Protein Powder

• 2 tsp. Vanilla Extract

• 1/4 tsp. Cream of Tartar

Filling

- 1 1/2 Cup Almond Flour

- 1 Tbsp. Cinnamon

- 1/2 Stick Butter

- 1/4 Cup Maple Syrup

- 1/4 Cup Erythritol

INSTRUCTION

1. Preheat your oven to 325F. If you're using a glass baking dish, use 300F.

2. Seperate the eggs from the egg whites for all 5 eggs. Cream together the egg yolks with 1/4 Cup Erythritol and 1/4 tsp. Liquid Stevia.

3. Once the egg yolks are creamed, add 6 Oz. Cream cheese and 1/4 Cup Unflavored Protein Powder. Mix this together well until a thick batter forms.

4. Beat your egg whites together with the 1/4 tsp. Cream of Tartar until stiff peaks form.

5. Fold the egg whites into the egg yolk mixture, doing 1/2 of the egg whites first and then the other half. Pour the batter into a round cake pan.

6. Mix together all of the "Filling" ingredients: 1 1/2 Cup Almond Flour, 1 Tbsp. Cinnamon, 1/2 Stick Butter, 1/4 Cup Maple Syrup , and 1/4 Cup Erythritol. This should form a "dough" of sorts. Take half and rip off little pieces to top the cake – push the pieces down if they don't sink on their own.

7. Bake for 20 minutes and then top with the rest of the cinnamon filling. Bake for another 20-30 minutes until a toothpick comes out clean. Let cool for 20 minutes before removing from the cake pan.

This will make 8 total slices of Ultimate Keto Coffee Cake, each slice coming out to 257 Calories, 26.7g Fats, 3.8g Net Carbs, and 12.8g Protein.

LOW CARB KEY LIME CHEESECAKES

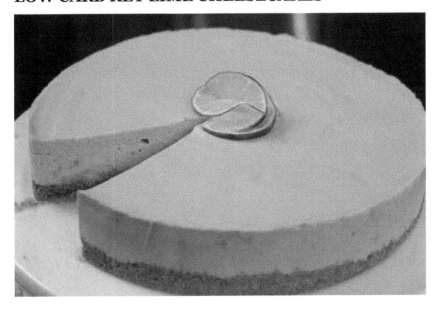

INGREDIENTS

Cheesecake Crust

- 1/2 cup Macadamia Nuts

- 1/2 cup Honeyville Almond Flour

- 1/4 cup Cold Butter

- 1/4 cup NOW Erythritol

- 1 large Egg Yolk

Key Lime Filling

- 8 oz. Cream Cheese

- 1/4 cup Butter

- 1/4 cup NOW Erythritol

- 1/4 tsp. Liquid Stevia

- 1-2 tbsp. Key Lime Juice (about 2 Key Limes – fresh is best)

- 2 large Eggs

- Zest of 2 Key Limes

INSTRUCTION

1. Preheat your oven to 350F. In a food processor, add the 1/2 cup of maca-damia nuts.

2. Grind the nuts into a coarse meal consistency, then add 1/4 cup of NOW erythritol.

3. Pulse for a few moments and then add 1/2 Cup Honeyville almond flour.

4. Pulse again until all is combined.

5. Cube 1/4 cup cold butter and add that into the food processor. Pulse again until the mixture starts to clump.

6. Add 1 egg yolk and pulse again until all of the dough clumps.

7. Remove the dough from the food processor and knead together with your hands.

8. Using some silicone cupcake molds (or just a regular greased cupcake tin), fill the wells about 1/8 to 1/4 of the way full. This depends on how thick you like your crust. If you make the crust thin, you will be able to make more cheesecake cupcakes.

9. Bake the crust for 5-7 minutes at 350F. They shouldn't be browned when you take them out, they will look greasy and undercooked.

10. While the crust is cooking, beat together 1 block of cream cheese (8 oz.) and 1/4 cup butter.

11. Once the butter and cream cheese is combined, add the 2 eggs and mix again.

12. Add 1/4 Cup NOW erythritol and 1/4 tsp. liquid stevia then mix again.

13. Finally, add the zest of about 2 key limes and the juice from 2 (this is about 2 Tbsp. of juice). Mix again until fully combined.

14. Once the crusts are out of the oven, let them cool for 3-5 minutes and then pour the mixture into the molds. Fill them so they leave some space at the top because they will rise as they cook and can spill over.

15. Bake the cheesecakes for 30-35 minutes at 350F.

16. Cool the cheesecakes for 20-30 minutes and then store in the fridge over-night.

17. Add some extra key lime zest over the top and serve!

This makes 12 total Key Lime Cheesecakes.

Each cheesecake has 226 Calories, 20.8g Fats, 2.2g Net Carbs, and 4.2g Protein.

CARAMEL POTS DE CRÈM

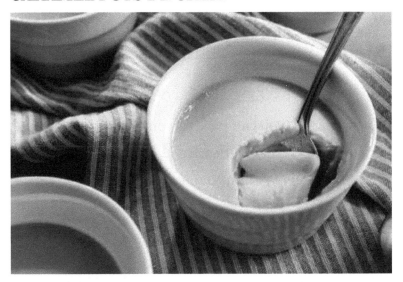

INGREDIENTS

- 1 1/2 cup Heavy Cream

- 1/4 cup NOW Erythritol (powdered)

- 1/4 tsp. Liquid Stevia

- 1/4 tsp. Salt

- 4 large Egg Yolks

- 6 tbsp. Water

- 1 tbsp. Maple Syrup (sub in 1 tsp. Maple Extract + 1/4 tsp. Xanthan Gum if you'd like)

- 1/2 tsp. Vanilla Extract

- 1 tsp. Maple Extract

INSTRUCTION

1. Preheat your oven to 300F. Start by separating the yolks of 4 eggs and setting them aside. You can save the whites to add to different cake recipes around the site.

2. Using a spice grinder (you can pick this one up cheap), powder 1/4 cup NOW erythritol. Be careful when you take the lid off because powder will float into the air.

3. Mix the powdered erythritol with 6 tbsp. water in a small saucepan.

4. Mix together 1 1/2 cups heavy cream, 1/4 tsp. liquid stevia, 1/4 tsp. salt, 1/2 tsp. vanilla extract, and 1 tsp. maple extract in a bigger saucepan.

5. Bright both of the mixtures to a rolling boil. Once the cream reaches a boil, stir vigorously and turn heat down to low. Occasionally stir this as you work with the other mixture.

6. Once the water and erythritol has been boiling for a minute, add 1 tbsp. maple syrup. If you don't want to make the whole maple syrup recipe for 1 tbsp., you're welcome to sub in 1 tsp. Maple Extract + 1/4 tsp. Xanthan Gum if you'd like.

7. Whisk egg yolks well with a whisk until lighter in color.

8. Continue boiling the water and erythritol mixture until it has reduced some and a watery syrup is formed.

9. Pour the water and erythritol mixture into the heavy cream and stir to combine.

10. Slowly pour 1/4 of the cream mixture into the egg yolks while mixing. You want to temper the egg yolks so make sure you add slowly and not too much at once.

11. Measure out the mixture between 4 or 6 ramekins depending on the size of the ramekin.

12. Fill baking sheet 2/3 of the way with water. Put your ramekins in the water and bake at 300F for 40 minutes.

13. Take out of the oven and let cool for 10-15 minutes. You can not refrigerate them if you'd like them to be more of a light custard or pudding texture. You can eat them warm for a velvety soft and smooth texture.

14. Who are we kidding? Serve them up!

This made 4 servings, but you are welcome to divide them into smaller servings.

Each serving was 359 Calories, 34.9g Fats, 3g Net Carbs, and 2.8g Protein.

PECAN BUTTER CHIA SEED BLONDIES

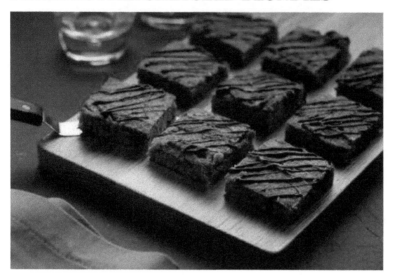

INGREDIENTS

- 2 1/4 cups Pecans, roasted

- 1/2 cup Chia Seeds, ground

- 1/4 cup Butter, melted

- 1/4 cup Erythritol, powdered

- 3 tbsp. SF Torani Salted

Caramel

- 10 drops Liquid Stevia

- 3 large Eggs

- 1 tsp. Baking Powder

• 3 tbsp. Heavy Cream

• 1 pinch Salt

INSTRUCTION

1. Preheat oven to 350F. Measure out 2 1/4 cup pecans and bake for about 10 minutes. Once you can smell a nutty aroma,remove nuts and set aside.

2. Grind 1/2 cup whole chia seeds in a spice grinder until a meal forms.

3. Remove chia meal and place in a bowl. Next, grind 1/4 cup Erythritol in a spice grinder until powdered. Set in the same bowl as the chia meal.

4. Place 2/3 of roasted pecans in food processor.

5. Process nuts, scraping sides down as needed, until a smooth nut butter is

formed.

6. Add 3 large eggs, 10 drops liquid stevia, 3 tbsp. SF Salted Caramel Torani Syrup, and a pinch of salt to the chia mixture. Mix this together well.

7. Add pecan butter to the batter and mix again.

8. Using a rolling pin, smash the rest of the roasted pecans into chunks inside of a plastic bag.

9. Add crushed pecans and 1/4 cup melted butter into the batter.

10. Mix batter well, then add 3 tbsp. Heavy cream and 1 tsp. Baking Powder. Mix everything together well.

11. Measure out the batter into a 9×9 tray and smooth out.

12. Bake for 20 minutes or until desired consistency.

13. Let cool for about 10 minutes. Slice off the edges of the brownie to create a uniform square. This is what I call "the bakers treat" – yep, you guessed it!

14. Snack on those bad boys while you get them ready to serve to everyone else. The so-called "best part" of the brownie are the edges, and that's why you deserve to have all of it.

15. Serve up and eat to your hearts (or rather macros) content!

 This makes 16 total Pecan Butter Chia Seed Blondies.

Each blondie comes out to 174 Calories, 17.1g Fats, 1.1g Net Carbs, and 3.9g Protein.

KETO PUMPKIN SNICKERDOODLE COOKIES

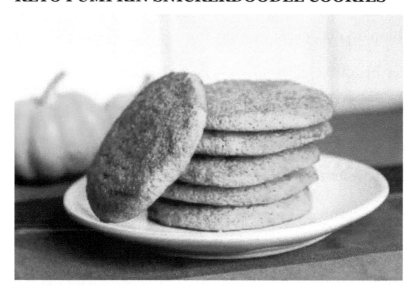

INGREDIENTS

The Cookies

• 1 1/2 cups Almond Flour

• 1/4 cup Butter, salted

• 1/2 cup Pumpkin Puree

• 1 tsp. Vanilla Extract

• 1/2 tsp. Baking Powder

• 1 large Egg

• 1/4 cup Erythritol

• 25 drops Liquid Stevia

The Topping

• 1 tsp. Pumpkin Pie Spice

• 2 tsp. Erythritol

INSTRUCTION

1. Pre-heat oven to 350F. Measure out almond flour, erythritol, and baking powder then mix together well.

2. Secondly, measure out the butter, pumpkin puree, vanilla, and liquid ste- via in a separate container.

3. Microwave mixture if needed for easier mixing. Add all wet ingredients (including the egg) to the almond flour and erythritol.

4. Mix everything together well until a pasty dough is formed.

5. Roll the dough into small balls and set on a cookie sheet covered with a

silpat. You should have about 15 cookies in total.

6. Press the balls flat with your hand (or the bottom side of a jar) and bake for 12-13 minutes.

7. While the cookies are cooking, run 2 tsp. erythritol and 1 tsp. pumpkin pie spice through a spice grinder to powder the erythritol.

8. Once the cookies are out of the oven, sprinkle with the topping and let cool completely.

This makes a total of 15 Keto Pumpkin Snickerdoodle Cookies.

Per cookie, they are 99 Calories, 8.9g Fats, 1.7g Net Carbs, and 2.9g Protein.

FRIED QUESO FRESCO

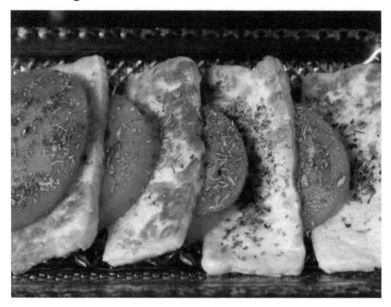

INGREDIENTS

• 1 lb. Queso Fresco

• 1 Tbsp. Coconut Oil

• 1/2 Tbsp. Olive Oil

INSTRUCTION

1. Grab your queso fresco. I am using 1 pound but the serving sizes is to your own needs.

2. Chop your queso fresco. You can either use cubes or rectangles. It all de-

pends on your own preference. I personally think rectangles turn out better.

3. Heat 1 Tbsp. Coconut Oil and 1/2 Tbsp. Olive Oil in a pan on high. Bring

this to the smoke point.

4. Right as the oil hits the smoke point, add your cheese.

5. Let the cheese cook on one side, flip it over to the other side and contin-

ue cooking.

6. If you're cooking cubed cheese, you will need to cook in on each side.

7. Remove the cheese from the pan and rest on paper towels to cool and

drain off excess oil.

Per serving, it is 243 Calories, 19.5g Fats, 0g Net Carbs, and 16g Protein.

RED PEPPER SPINACH SALAD

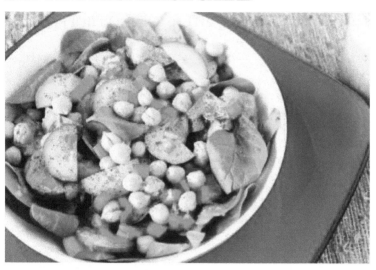

INGREDIENTS

- 6 Cups Spinach

- 1/4 Cup Ranch Dressing

- 3 Tbsp. Parmesan Cheese

- 1 tsp. Red Pepper Flakes

INSTRUCTION

1. In a large mixing bowl, measure out 6 Cup of Spinach.

2. Add 1/4 Cup Ranch Dressing and mix it into the spinach. Then, add 3 Tbsp. Parmesan Cheese and 1 tsp. Red Pepper Flakes. Mix well again.

3. Serve as a side salad.

Per serving, you are looking at: 208 Calories, 18g Fats, 3.5g Net Carbs, and 8g Protein.

BACON INFUSED SUGAR SNAP PEAS

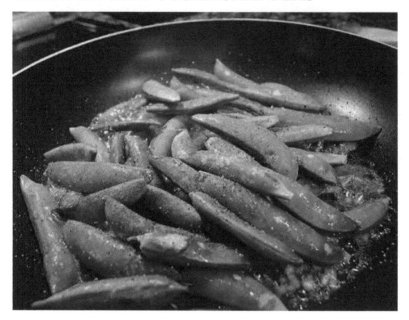

INGREDIENTS

- 3 Cups Sugar Snap Peas (~200g)

- 1/2 Lemon Juice

- 3 Tbsp. Bacon Fat

- 2 tsp. Garlic

- 1/2 tsp. Red Pepper Flakes

INSTRUCTION

1. Add 3 Tbsp. Bacon Fat to a pan and bring to it's smoking point.

2. Once the bacon fat is at the smoking point, add 2 tsp. Garlic. Reduce the heat of the pan to medium and let this cook for 1-2 minutes, until the garlic is browned.

3. Add 3 Cups of Sugar Snap Peas to the pan and let this cook for a moment.

4. Add the juice of 1/2 lemon over the Sugar Snap Peas.

5. Let this cook for 1-2 minutes.

6. Remove and serve. Garnish with red pepper flakes and lemon zest.

Per Serving, you're looking at: 147 Calories, 13.3g Fats, 4.3g Net Carbs, and 1.3g Protein.

BACON JAMMIN' GREEN BEANS

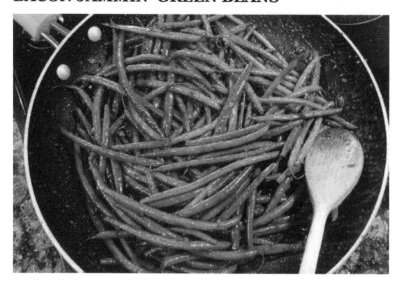

INGREDIENTS

• 2 1/2 Cups Fresh Green Beans (~425g)

• 3 Tbsp. Bacon Jam

• 1 Tbsp. Olive Oil

INSTRUCTION

1. Have your green beans ready to go.

2. Bring water to a rolling boil in a pan on the stove.

3. Add your green beans to the pan and let boil for 3-4 minutes.

4. Drain your green beans and add them to an ice bath to blanch them. This

stops the cooking process and helps keep their crispness.

5. In a skillet, add 3 Tbsp. Bacon Jam and 1 Tbsp. Olive Oil.

6. Drain your green beans and put them on a kitchen towel to dry. Bring your bacon jam and olive oil to a sizzle.

7. Add your green beans to the pan.

8. Stir everything well and cook for 1-2 minutes.

9. Serve green beans while warm.

Per Serving, they have: 112 Calories, 6.6g Fats, 5.5g Net Carbs, and 5.2g Protein

ROASTED PECAN GREEN BEAN

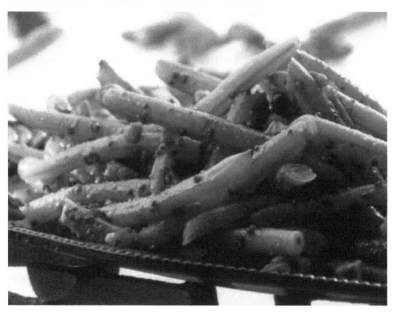

INGREDIENTS

- 1 lb. Green Beans

- 1/4 Cup Olive Oil

- 1/2 Cup Chopped Pecans

- 1/4 Cup Parmesan Cheese

- 1 Lemon's Zest

- 2 tsp. Minced Garlic

- 1 tsp. Red Pepper Flakes

INSTRUCTION

1. Preheat your oven to 450F, then empty your green beans into a large mixing bowl.

2. Add 1/4 Cup Pecans into a food processor. If you don't have a food processor, I highly recommend getting one – I use this one, that's $30.

3. Grind the pecans in the food processor until your desired consistency is reached. Some pieces should be small and crumbly, others should be larger adding contrasting textures.

4. Add 1/4 Cup Olive Oil, 1/4 Cup Parmesan Cheese, the Zest of 1 Lemon, 2 tsp. Minced Garlic, and 1 tsp. Red Pepper Flakes to the green beans.

5. Using a fork (or better yet, your hands), mix together the green beans and the rest of the ingredients.

6. Add foil to a baking sheet, then spread your green beans onto the baking sheet. Don't worry if some are sitting on top of the others, it will give more textural contrast throughout the whole dish.

7. Roast the green beans for 20-25 minutes (depending on how your oven is). Make sure you keep an eye on them after the 20 minute mark.

8. Let cool for 4-5 minutes and then serve!

This makes 4 total servings, each serving being 273 Calories, 25.3g Fats, 5g Net Carbs, and 5.5g Protein

BOK CHOY CHICKEN RECIPE

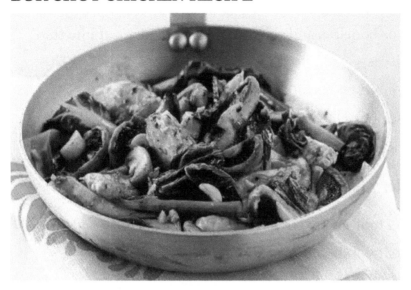

Bok Choy Chicken – easy vegetable stir-fry recipe with bok choy, chicken, garlic and a simple sauce. So EASY, healthy and takes only 15 minutes.

Prep Time 10 minutes

Cook Time 10 minutes

Total Time 20 minutes

Servings 2 people

Calories 188 kcal

Ingredients

- 6 oz boneless and skinless chicken breast, cut into thin pieces
- 2 tablespoons oil
- 8 oz bok choy, sliced into pieces
- 1 inch piece ginger, peeled and sliced into pieces

Marinade:

- 1/2 tablespoon soy sauce
- 1/2 tablespoon cornstarch

Sauce:

- 1/2 tablespoon oyster sauce
- 2 tablespoons water
- 1/4 teaspoon sesame oil
- 3 dashes white pepper
- 1 teaspoon wine
- 1/2 teaspoon sugar

Instructions

1. Marinate the chicken with the ingredients in Marinade for 10 minutes. Combine all the ingredients in the Sauce in a small bowl, stir to blend well.

2. Heat 1/2 tablespoon oil in a wok until the oil becomes hot. Add the chicken and quickly stir-fry until the surface of the chicken turn opaque or white. Dish out and set aside. This step seals in the juice in the chicken so the texture is tender and vevelty smooth.

3. Heat up the remaining oil in the wok until hot. Add the ginger into the wok and stir-fry until aromatic. Add the chicken back into the wok and do a few quick stirs. Add in the bok choy and stir to combine well. Transfer the sauce into the wok and continue to stir-fry until the bok choy is cooked but remain crisp. Do not overcook.

4. Dish out and serve immediately with steamed white rice.

Nutrition Facts

Amount Per Serving (2 people)

Calories 188

Total Fat 16g 25%

Total Carbohydrates 2.5g 1%

Sugars 1.3g

Protein 19.7g 39%

GARLIC BUTTER STEAK RECIPE

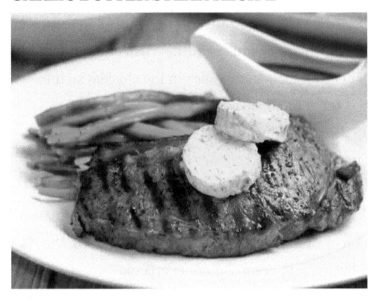

Garlic Butter Steak - juicy and tender steak cooked in a cast-iron skillet. Topped with compound garlic butter, this skillet steak recipe is so easy and delicious!

Prep Time 5 minutes

Cook Time 15 minutes

Total Time 20 minutes

Servings 4 people

Calories 248 kcal

Ingredients

- 2 12-oz top sirloin steaks (about 1 1/2-inch thick steak)
- coarse salt
- ground black pepper
- 1 tablespoon vegetable oil
- Garlic Butter
- 2 tablespoons salted butter, softened
- 2 cloves garlic, minced
- 1 tablespoon chopped parsley

Instructions

1. Season both sides of the top sirloin steaks generously with salt and ground black pepper. Set aside.
2. Top Sirloin Steak
3. Prepare the Garlic Butter by mixing the butter, garlic and parsley together. Let cool in the fridge.
4. Garlic Butter
5. Heat up a cast-iron skillet on high heat until smoking hot. Add the oil. Transfer the steak to the skillet and pan-sear each side (do not turn) for about 4 minutes. Turn over and pan-sear the other side for another 4 minutes. Transfer the steak to a serving platter.
6. Add a dollop of the Garlic Butter on top of the steak and serve immediately.

Nutrition Facts

Amount Per Serving

Calories 248

Total Fat 9g 14%

Protein 38g 76%

Calcium 4%

PARMESAN GARLIC BREAD RECIPE

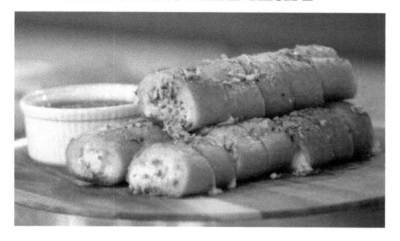

Parmesan Garlic Bread - Turn regular French bread into delicious, buttery parmesan garlic bread with this quick and easy recipe.

Prep Time 10 minutes

Cook Time 15 minutes

Total Time 25 minutes

Servings 3 people

Ingredients

- 1 loaf crusty country-style french bread
- 1 1/4 sticks salted butter, melted
- 5 cloves garlic, pureed or very finely chopped

- 5 tablespoons bottled Parmesan cheese
- 1 teaspoon finely chopped parsley leaves

Instructions

1. Preheat the overn to 375F. Slice the horizontally into halves. Set aside.
2. In a small bowl, combine the melted butter, garlic, Parmesan cheese and parsley together. Stir to mix well. Brush the mixture generously on the sliced French bread.
3. Bake for 15 minutes or until the garlic Parmesan mixture is a bit crusty. Remove from heat, let cool a little bit, and slice into pieces using bread knife. It's best served warm.

Nutrition Facts

Calories 663

Total Fat 43g 66%

Total Carbohydrates 77g 26%

Sugars 4g

Protein 19g 38%

GINGER SOY BOK CHOY RECIPE

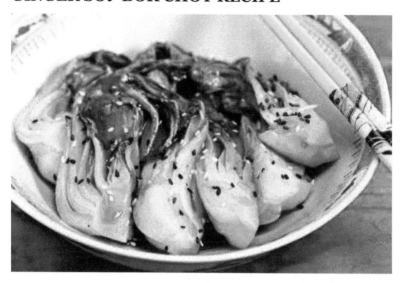

Ginger Soy Bok Choy - the easiest and healthiest bok choy recipe ever. Calls for only 5 ingredients and 10 minutes to make. It's so delicious.

Prep Time 5 minutes

Cook Time 5 minutes

Total Time 10 minutes

Servings 2 people

Calories 94 kcal

Ingredients

- 1 tablespoons oil
- 2- inch piece ginger, peeled and minced
- 12 oz. baby bok choy
- 1 tablespoon soy sauce
- 1 teaspoon lemon juice

Instructions

1. Rinse the bok choy with cold water, drained. Cut and remove the lower part of the bok choy stems.
2. Cut the (bigger) leaves lengthwise to halves. Set aside.
3. Heat up a skillet with the oil. Saute the ginger until aromatic, add the bok choy.
4. Stir fry and toss quickly a few times before adding the soy sauce and lemon juice.
5. As soon as the bok choy are wilted, dish out and serve immediately.
6. DO NOT OVERCOOK.

Nutrition Facts

Total Fat 7g 11%

Total Carbohydrates 5g 2%

Sugars 2g

Protein 2g 4%

ASIAN-BRINED PORK CHOPS RECIPE

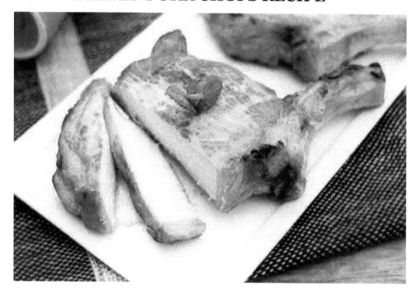

Asian-brined Pork Chops - flavorful and delicious Asian pork chops, so easy to make dinner is ready in 30 mins.

Prep Time 10 minutes

Cook Time 10 minutes

Marinade Time 2 hours

Total Time 20 minutes

Servings 4 people

Ingredients:

- 4 bone-in pork chops, 3/4-inch thick
- 1/8 teaspoon salt or to taste
- 1 tablespoon cooking oil
- Brine:
- 3/4 cup mirin
- 1/2 cup low sodium soy sauce
- 3 ounces fresh ginger, thinly sliced
- 6-8 small dried chilies
- 1 orange, thinly sliced
- 1 1/2 tablespoons sesame oil
- 1 1/2 cups cold water
- Garnish (optional):
- Mint leaves

Instructions

1. Lightly season the pork chops with the salt.
2. Mix all the ingredients for the Brine in a container or pot, just big enough for the pork chops. Marinade the pork chops in the Brine for at least 2 hours or best overnight.
3. Before cooking, remove the pork chops from the Brine and let them come to room temperature. Pat the pork chops dry with paper towels.

4. Heat the cooking oil in a non-stick skillet on medium heat.

    Pan-fry the pork chops for about 4-5 minutes each side. Transfer and wrap the pork chops with foil. Let them rest for 8-10 minutes before serving.

Recipe Notes

You can choose to use boneless pork chops. Adjust your cooking time accordingly.

Nutrition Facts

Calories 482

Total Fat 24g 37%

Total Carbohydrates 29g 10%

Protein 38g 76%

GARLIC NOODLES RECIPE

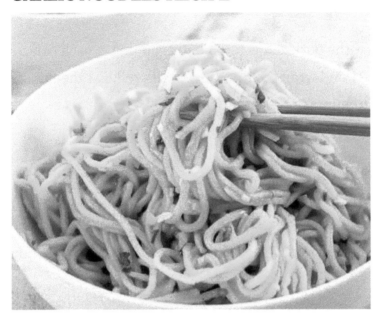

Garlic Noodles - The easiest and best noodles with garlic, butter, Parmesan cheese and Asian seasoning sauces. Tastes just like the best Asian restaurants!

Prep Time 15 minutes

Cook Time 5 minutes

Total Time 20 minutes

Servings 5 people

Ingredients:

- 20 oz yellow noodles or spaghetti
- 1 tablespoon bottled grated Parmesan cheese
- water, for boiling the noodles

Garlic Sauce:

- 1 stick unsalted butter (4 oz/110 g/1/2 cup/8 tablespoons)
- 2 tablespoons minced garlic, or more to taste
- 1 tablespoon Maggie seasoning sauce
- 1 tablespoon oyster sauce
- 1 tablespoon fish sauce
- 1 tablespoon sugar

Instructions

1. Rinse the yellow noodles with running water to discard the oil from the noodles. Drain and set aside.
2. Heat up a pot of water until boiling. Add the noodles into the boiling water and cook the noodles until al dente (you want it to still have a good chewy bite), or for a few minutes. You can taste the texture of the noodles while cooking. Do not overcook as the noodles will turn soggy. Transfer the noodles out and drain dry.

3. Prepare the garlic sauce using a saute pan on medium to low heat. Add the butter into the pan and when it melts, add the garlic and saute until aromatic but not browned. Add all the seasonings into the pan, stir to combine well. Transfer the garlic sauce into a small bowl.
4. To serve, just toss all the noodles with the garlic sauce. Add the cheese, toss to combine well. Serve immediately.

Recipe Notes

For individual serving of the garlic noodles, take some noodles to a bowl and add some garlic sauce to taste. Drizzle some grated Parmesan cheese, stir to combine well before serving. If you can't find any yellow noodles, you can use spaghetti or linguine.

Nutrition Facts

Amount Per Serving (5 people)

Calories 604

Total Fat 20g 31%

Total Carbohydrates 88g 29%

Protein 15g 30%

CINNAMON ROLL "OATMEAL"

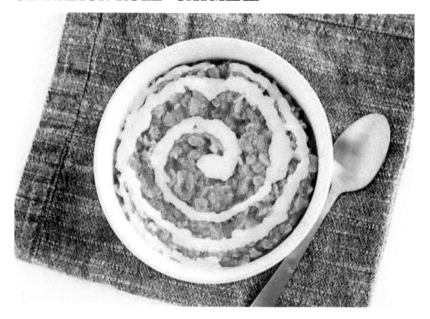

INGREDIENTS

• 1 cup Crushed Pecans

• 1/3 cup Flax Seed Meal

• 1/3 cup Chia Seeds

• 1/2 cup Cauliflower, riced (~ 3 oz.)

• 3 1/2 cups Coconut Milk

• 1/4 cup Heavy Cream

• 3 oz. Cream Cheese

• 3 tbsp. Butter

• 1 1/2 tsp. Cinnamon

197

- 1 tsp. Maple Flavor

- 1/2 tsp. Vanilla

- 1/4 tsp. Nutmeg

- 1/4 tsp. Allspice

- 3 tbsp. Erythritol, powdered

- 10-15 drops Liquid Stevia

- 1/8 tsp. Xanthan Gum (optional)

INSTRUCTION

1. Measure out chia seeds and 1/3 cup flax seeds (ground) and set aside.

2. Rice 1/2 cup of cauliflower in a food processor. Set aside for a moment.

3. Add 1 cup raw pecans to a ziploc bag and use a rolling pin to crush them.

4. Make sure they're not too small, because you want them to add texture to

the dish.

5. Add pecans to a pan over low heat to toast.

6. In a saucepan, heat 3 1/2 cups coconut milk. Once warm, add cauliflower

and continue to cook until it starts to boil.

7. Turn the heat down to medium-low and add your seasonings: 1 1/2 tsp.

cinnamon, 1 tsp. maple flavor, 1/2 tsp. vanilla, 1/4 tsp. Nutmeg, and 1/4 tsp.

Allspice.

8. In a spice grinder, grind 3 tbsp. erythritol until it is completely powdered.

9. Add erythritol and 10-15 drops liquid stevia to the pan and stir in well.

10. Add the flaxseed meal and chia seed to the pan and mix well. This will start to thicken tremendously.

11. Measure out 1/4 cup heavy cream, 3 tbsp. butter, and 3 oz. Cream Cheese.

12. Once your mixture is hot again, add the toasted pecans, cream, butter, and cream cheese. Mix together well. Here, you can add 1/8 tsp. xanthan gum if you would like it to be a bit thicker. Enjoy!

Each serving comes out to be 398 Calories, 37.7g Fats, 3.1g Net Carbs, and 8.8g Protein.

ROASTED ASPARAGUS WITH GARLIC RECIPE

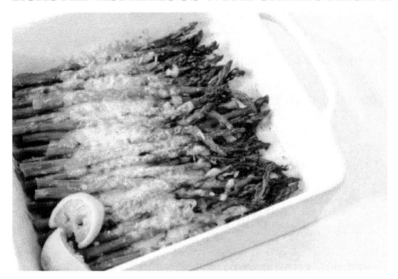

Garlic Roasted Asparagus - healthy oven baked asparagus with garlic. This recipe takes 4 ingredients and only 12 mins to make this quick and easy side dish.

Prep Time 5 minutes

Cook Time 12 minutes

Total Time 17 minutes

Servings 3 people

Ingredients

- 1 lb asparagus, bottom stems trimmed
- 2 tablespoons melted salted butter
- 1 pinch salt
- 3 cloves garlic, thinly sliced

Instructions

1. Preheat oven to 400 F.
2. In a sheet pan, toss the asparagus with the melted butter. Season the asparagus with a good pinch of salt.
3. Arrange the garlic slices on top of the asparagus.
4. Roast the asparagus for 12 minutes. Remove from oven and serve immediately.

Nutrition Facts

Amount Per Serving (3 people)

Calories 98

Total Fat 7g 11%

Total Carbohydrates 6g 2%

Protein 3g 6%

BAKED CHICKEN AND POTATO CASSEROLE RECIPE

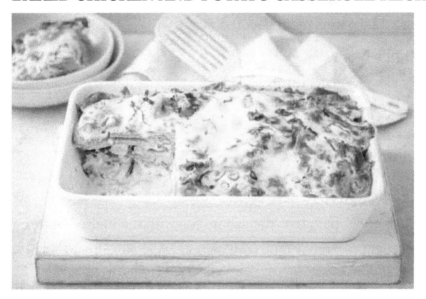

Baked Chicken and Potato Casserole - crazy delicious and easy chicken potato casserole recipe loaded with potatoes, cheddar cheese, bacon and cream.

Prep Time 10 minutes

Cook Time 1 hour 30 minutes

Total Time 1 hour 40 minutes

Servings 2 people

Ingredients

- 1/4 teaspoon salt or to taste
- 1/2 teaspoon sugar
- 3 dashes ground black pepper
- 1/4 cup heavy whipping cream
- 2 medium-sized potatoes, peeled and cut into pieces
- 8 oz boneless, skinless chicken breasts, cut into cubes
- 2 slices Canadian bacon, cut into pieces
- 4 tablespoons unsalted butter, cut into small pieces
- 1 cup shredded cheddar cheese
- 1 stalk scallion, green part only, cut into small rounds

Instructions

1. Heat oven to 350 degrees F. Lightly grease a 9" x 9" baking pan with some oil or butter.
2. Add the salt, sugar, and pepper to the heavy whipping cream. Lightly stir to combine well.
3. Spread the potatoes, follow by the chicken, in one single layer.
4. Sprinkle the bacon, butter, and then top with half of the cheddar cheese and the scallions.
5. Pour the heavy cream over top of casserole. Cover with aluminum foil and bake for 1 hour. Uncover the pan and bake for another 30 minutes. In the last 10 minutes, sprinkle with the

remaining cheddar cheese and bake until the cheese is slightly crusty. Remove from the oven and serve immediately.

Recipe Notes

Instead of Canadian bacon, you can use 1 or 2 strips of bacon. If you use bacon, pre-cooked them until they are crisp first.

Nutrition Facts

Amount Per Serving (2 people)

Calories 385

Total Fat 64g 98%

Potassium 1440mg 41%

Total Carbohydrates 31g 10%

Protein 48g 96%

ITALIAN SHRIMP PASTA RECIPE

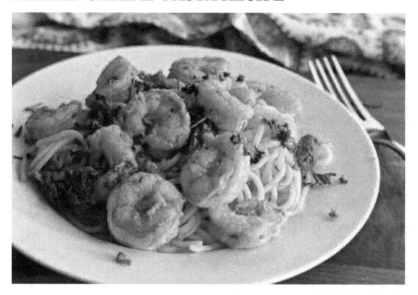

This is a proper Italian Shrimp Pasta recipe, the authentic way Italian home cooks and chefs make shrimp pasta. The pasta is fresh, healthy, with an absolutely mouthwatering homemade tomato sauce.

Prep Time 10 minutes

Cook Time 10 minutes

Total Time 20 minutes

Servings 2 people

Ingredients

- 4 oz spaghetti pasta
- 2 tablespoons extra virgin olive oil
- 3 cloves garlic, finely minced
- 4 oz Campari tomatoes, cut into thin wedges
- 1/4 cup chicken broth
- 1/2 teaspoon chicken bouillon
- 4 oz peeled and deveined shrimp or jumbo prawn, butterflied
- 3/4 teaspoon salt or more to taste
- freshly ground black pepper
- 1 teaspoon chopped Italian parsley

Instructions

1. Bring a pot of salted water to boil. Cook the spaghetti al dente, according to package instruction.
2. In a skillet or pan on medium-low heat, add the extra virgin olive oil. Saute the garlic until sizzling but not browned. Add the tomatoes, chicken broth and chicken bouillon. As soon as it bubbles, add the shrimp. Cook and stir until the shrimps are cooked and the tomatoes break down.

3. Add the spaghetti, salt and generous dose of freshly ground black pepper. Stir to combine well. Turn off the heat.
4. Top the Shrimp Pasta with chopped Italian parsley and serve immediately.

Nutrition Facts

Amount Per Serving (2 people)

Calories 392

Total Fat 15g 23%

Total Carbohydrates 46g 15%

Protein 16g 32%

GARLIC PARMESAN ROASTED CARROTS RECIPE

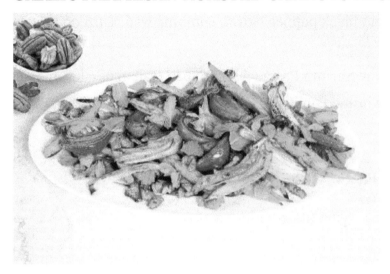

Garlic Parmesan Roasted Carrots - oven roasted carrots with butter, garlic and Parmesan cheese. The easiest and most delicious carrot recipes ever!

Prep Time 10 minutes

Cook Time 25 minutes

Total Time 35 minutes

Servings 2 people

Ingredients

1. 12 oz carrots, skin peeled
2. 2 tablespoons melted salted butter
3. 2 cloves garlic, minced
4. 3 tablespoons grated Parmesan cheese
5. 1 teaspoon chopped parsley

Instructions

1. Preheat the oven to 400F.
2. Mix the melted butter and garlic together. Coat the carrots well with the butter mixture.
3. Arrange the carrots on a baking sheet lined with parchment paper.
4. Drizzle the extra butter garlic mixture on top of the carrots. Roast for 15 minutes, then top the carrots with the Parmesan cheese.
5. Roast for another 10 minutes or until the cheese melts and slightly browned.
6. Remove from the oven and top with the parsley. Serve immediately.

Recipe Notes

For sweet versions of carrots, please try my honey butter roasted carrots, maple butter roasted baby carrots or candied carrots.

Nutrition Facts

Amount Per Serving (2 people)

Calories 186

Total Fat 14g 22%

Total Carbohydrates 18g 6%

Protein 5g 10%

GARLIC HERB GRILLED SALMON RECIPE

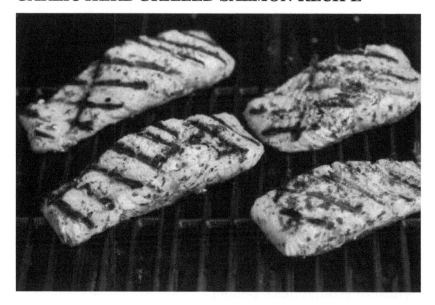

Garlic Herb Grilled Salmon - moist and juicy salmon with garlic, herbs, olive oil and lemon marinade. This is the best grilled salmon recipe ever and takes only 8 minutes on gas grill.

Prep Time 10 minutes

Cook Time 8 minutes

Marinade Time 20 minutes

Total Time 38 minutes

Servings 4 people

Ingredients

- 1 lb. salmon (top loin, loin or second cut)
- lemon wedges, for serving
- Marinade:
- 2 tablespoons olive oil
- 2 cloves garlic, minced
- 1 teaspoon chopped Italian basil
- 1 tablespoon chopped Italian parsley
- 1 tablespoon lemon juice
- 1/2 teaspoon salt
- 3 dashes ground black pepper

Instructions

1. Mix all the Marinade ingredients in a bowl, stir to mix well.
2. Marinate the salmon with the Marinade for 20 minutes.
3. Salmon fillet in grilled salmon marinade.
4. Heat up a gas grill to medium heat, at 350 degrees F. Remove the marinated salmon from the Marinade and place it on top of the gas grill. Place the salmon, skin side down at a 45 degree angle to form beautiful char marks. Grill the salmon for 4 minutes, uninterrupted. Turn the salmon over and grill for another 4 minutes,

uninterrupted. Baste with the remaining Marinade mixture while grilling.

5. Grilling salmon with skin on a gas grill.

Depending on the type of salmon cuts you use, you might need to grill it for longer (or shorter) time. The salmon is cooked when white stuff starts to seep out from the inside. If the salmon is not cooked yet but already charred, move the salmon to the indirect heat side of the gas grill. Cover the lid and cook for 1-2 minutes or until the inside is completely cooked through. Remove from the grill and serve immediately with lemon wedges, dill sauce, or sweet chili sauce.

Nutrition Facts

Amount Per Serving (4 people)

Calories 228

Total Fat 14g 22%

Total Carbohydrates 1g 0%

Protein 23g 46%

CONCLUSION

After an extensive research has been conducted, there is no doubt at all that The 5:2 diet involves eating normally for five days per week, then restricting your calorie intake to 500–600 calories on the other two days.

The 5:2 diet should be very effective for weight loss if done correctly. It may help reduce belly fat, as well as help maintain muscle mass during weight loss.

16:8 intermittent fasting is a popular form of intermittent fasting. Potential benefits include weight loss, fat loss, and a reduction in the risk of some diseases.

This diet plan may also be easier to follow than other types of fasting. People doing 16:8 intermittent fasting should focus on eating high fiber whole foods, and they should stay hydrated throughout the day.

The plan is not right for everyone. Individuals who wish to follow the 16:8 intermittent fasting diet should speak to a doctor or dietitian if they have any concerns or underlying health conditions.

Lightning Source UK Ltd.
Milton Keynes UK
UKHW020624140621
385475UK00001B/208